Caring for Children with HIV and AIDS

Edited by
**Rosie Claxton and
Tony Harrison**

Edward Arnold
A division of Hodder & Stoughton
LONDON MELBOURNE AUCKLAND

© 1991 Rosie Claxton, Tony Harrison

First published in Great Britain 1991

British Library Cataloguing in Publication Data

Caring for children with HIV infections and AIDS.
  I. Claxton, Rosie   II. Harrison, Tony
  616.970083

  ISBN 0–340–55256–5

Whilst the advice and information in this book is believed to be true and accurate at the date of going to press, neither the author nor the publisher can accept any legal responsibility or liability for any errors or omissions that may be made. In particular (but without limiting the generality of the preceding disclaimer) every effort has been made to check drug dosages; however, it is still possible that errors have been missed. Furthermore, dosage schedules are constantly being revised and new side effects recognised. For these reasons, the reader is strongly urged to consult the drug companies' printed instructions before administering any of the drugs recommended in this book.

Typeset by Wearside Tradespools, Boldon, Tyne and Wear.
Printed in Great Britain for Edward Arnold, a division of Hodder and Stoughton Limited, Mill Road, Dunton Green, Sevenoaks, Kent TN13 2YA by St Edmundsbury Press Limited, Bury St Edmunds, Suffolk and bound by Hartnolls Limited, Bodmin, Cornwall.

√ include in Bib?

Contents

Contributors

Janette Brierley, Director of Midwifery and Nursing Services, Women and Children's Health, East Surrey Health Authority, Redhill, Surrey. Formerly Midwifery Tutor, St. Mary's Hospital, Paddington, London.

Sheila Burns, Consultant Virologist, Regional Infectious Diseases Unit, City Hospital, Edinburgh.

Rosie Claxton, Health Adviser and HIV/AIDS Counsellor, Department of Genito-Urinary Medicine, Westminster Hospital, London.

John Cosgrove, Health Visitor, Forres Health Clinic, Forres, Morayshire. Formerly Specialist Health Visitor HIV/AIDS, City Hospital, Edinburgh.

Janet M. Hall, Senior Sister, Royal Alexandra Hospital for Sick Children, Brighton.

Tony Harrison, Nurse Teacher, Stockport, Tameside and Glossop College of Nursing, Stepping Hill Hospital, Stockport, Cheshire. Formerly Charge Nurse in Paediatric Medicine, Booth Hall Children's Hospital, Manchester.

Jim Kuykendall, HIV/AIDS Facilitator, Ealing, Hammersmith and Hounslow Family Health Services Authority, London. Formerly Lecturer in Psychology, AIDS Education Unit, Riverside College of Nursing, Charing Cross Hospital, London, and Child Life and Adolescent Specialist/ Counsellor, Paediatric Department, Charing Cross Hospital, London.

Rebekah Lwin, Principal Clinical Psychologist, Department of Psychological Medicine, The Hospitals for Sick Children, Great Ormond Street, London.

Susan Macqueen, Senior Nurse, Infection Control, The Hospitals for Sick Children, London.

Jacqueline Mok, Consultant Paediatrician, Department of Community Child Health and Regional Infectious Diseases Unit, City Hospital, Edinburgh, and part-time Senior Lecturer, Department of Child Life and Health, University of Edinburgh.

Marie-Louise Newell, Lecturer in Epidemiology, Institute of Child Health, University of London.

Catherine S. Peckham, Professor of Paediatric Epidemiology, Institute of Child Health, University of London.

Reg Pyne, Assistant Registrar, Standards and Ethics, United Kingdom Central Council for Nursing, Midwifery and Health Visiting, London.

Carolyn Roth, Senior Lecturer in Midwifery Studies, South Bank Polytechnic, London. Formerly Midwifery Tutor, St. Mary's Hospital, Paddington, London.

Kate Skinner, Lecturer in Social Work (Continuing Education), University of Stirling, Scotland.

Alex Susman-Shaw, Clinical Nurse Specialist, (Paediatric Haemophilia/ Haematology), Department of Haematology, Royal Manchester Childrens' Hospital, Pendlebury, Manchester.

Mark Winter, Director, Haemophilia Centre, Thanet District General Hospital, Margate, Kent.

Foreword

HIV affects everyone, and will continue to have an impact on the lives of all children. This important book is the first of its kind in the United Kingdom. In a rapidly developing field where knowledge is continually changing, this book provides a clear picture of the epidemiological and clinical aspects of HIV infection in children. There is an extensive and sensitive approach to the many other important issues which are part of the daily life for those living with HIV infection – for children, their families and their carers.

Rosie and Tony are to be congratulated for their commitment to raising awareness of paediatric HIV infection, both locally and internationally. This book is a reflection of their achievement.

I am delighted to have been involved with this book which will be of interest and value to all those who care for children and young people affected by HIV.

Candy Duggan
Nurse Counsellor
The Hospital for Sick Children
London
1991

Preface

There has been a spate of literature written about the effects of HIV (Human Immunodeficiency Virus) covering many facets of this new and challenging, tragic disease. However one notable void in the published work is in the field of paediatric HIV disease, together with its ramifications. It could be argued that the number of children known to be infected in the Western world is still relatively low, hence the scanty amount of reference material available.

The aim of this book is to create an awareness of the disease, and provide a broad overview of some of the issues and problems encountered by those who have pioneered the work involved in caring for families and children living with HIV and AIDS (Acquired Immune Deficiency Syndrome). The text is not solely theoretical or academic. The contributors have valuable personal and professional experience from which knowledge and understanding have developed.

The text is non-prescriptive and there is a deliberate intention to avoid any moral or judgemental bias. Each chapter has been devised to 'stand alone': the experiences of each author are different. The whole work demonstrates the need for team-work and a multi-disciplinary approach in providing care. Many contributors have highlighted similar issues from individual view-points. This illustrates the need for emphasising the importance of some of the common threads within the book.

The somewhat clinical nature of the text echoes the pattern of the lives of those affected by the disease; those living with HIV and AIDS have had to adjust to a 'medical' way of life. The chronic and steady progression of the illness dictates the need for appropriate nursing and clinical intervention, linking with social and emotional support. However it must always be remembered that individuals – adults and children, wherever possible, should be given the choice and power to control all decisions made affecting their lives, including the care they receive.

At the time of writing most of the studies of children with HIV infection are retrospective. Research and information pertaining to treatment, whether clinical, psychological or social, is at an embryonic stage, and there are ethical, economical and political dilemmas involved. The issues of preparation and planning care for families where HIV is a multi-generational problem are complex and will tax those making policies and provisions both in hospitals and the community.

This text is not definitive; there are many issues yet to be discussed. For example, caring for a family with differing needs in a single setting: perhaps a mother with HIV-related memory loss, together with her child affected by a chronic lung disorder caused by HIV. There are areas of concern for children who may be required to undergo a test for HIV infection prior to receiving surgery, and there will be concern too relating to organ donation and HIV. These suggestions and many others will continue to challenge those involved at all levels of health care provision. As time progresses and the disease presents new problems there will be a need for further debate. In the immediate future, all those involved in health and social care will have to treat each individual's problem with discretion, using sound professional judgement, to enable those living with HIV to receive the best possible care at all times.

It is hoped that this book will be of value to a wide readership. Although the origins of the book stem from a nursing context, the need for a multidisciplinary approach is amply proven.

Wherever there are children, the possibility of HIV infection may need consideration. The settings involving children and families are diverse and range from places of custodial care to all agencies providing educational and other care for children, as well as centres of paediatric excellence. It is hoped that this text will provide useful information whenever the reader is involved in caring for children and their families.

Rosie Claxton
1991

Acknowledgements

There are many who have shown interest and given us support in the preparation of this book. Firstly, our gratitude must go to all the contributors who have given very generously of their time and energy.

Secondly, and no less importantly, we owe much to those children and adults whose lives have been changed by this tragic illness. For those we know, and those farther afield – we wish that there had never been a need to write this book.

Our thanks and appreciation are due to the many others who have given us encouragement and help – our friends, our families and our colleagues. It is important that they should be acknowledged together with Sue Burr, Candy Duggan, Ben Thomas, Gordon Flintham, Carol Lindsay-Smith, Peter Vickers, Barbara Weller and, in particular, Nancy Loffler.

Rosie Claxton
Tony Harrison
1991

1 Epidemiology of paediatric HIV infection

Marie-Louise Newell and Catherine S. Peckham

Human Immunodeficiency Virus (HIV) is the virus that causes Acquired Immunodeficiency Syndrome (AIDS). Infection can be acquired through:

- penetrative sex with an infected person
- transfusion of infected blood or blood products, or the sharing of contaminated needles and syringes
- from semen donation, and tissue and donor transplants
- from an infected mother to her child during pregnancy or in the perinatal period (known as vertical or perinatal transmission).

Although HIV has been found in saliva, sweat, tears and urine, there is no evidence that HIV can be acquired from these sources. Indeed, it is important to stress that infection has not been transmitted by the following:

- casual contact with an infected person
- droplets coughed or sneezed into the air
- the sharing of utensils such as cups and plates
- swimming pools
- toilet seats
- insects.

Information on the lack of casual transmission from children to their close household contacts is accumulating and there have been no reports of transmission of HIV acquired from children in family, day or foster-care settings, or schools[1,2,3].

Precautions taken to prevent the spread of Hepatitis B virus, which is much more infectious than HIV, are more than adequate to prevent transmission of HIV[4,5,6,7]. The exclusion of donors at increased risk of HIV infection and the testing of donated blood for HIV now virtually eliminate the risk of infection from blood or blood products[8]. (See also Chapter 4, Part 1 with regard to Haemophilia.) Testing of blood in the UK was introduced in 1985, but in countries where testing is not routine blood remains an important source of infection and the use of blood and blood products should be restricted. Similarly, in many countries organ, semen and breastmilk donors are also screened for HIV infection.

Little is known about factors which influence transmission of infection. Biological co-factors which enhance the transmission of HIV by sexual contact have been identified in several studies, and people with genital lesions due to other sexually transmitted diseases appear to be both more efficient transmitters of and more susceptible to HIV infection[9]. Studies suggest that male-to-female transmission is more efficient than female-to-male transmission, but larger numbers are required before definitive statements can be

1

made. There is increasing evidence to suggest that clinical status influences the rate of transmission, and people who are HIV symptomatic may be more infectious. However, at present the biological variables which determine both infectivity and susceptibility are incompletely understood[10].

The AIDS epidemic

AIDS was first described in adults in 1982 in the USA and was first recognised in children in 1983 by Rubenstein in New York[11]. The causative agent, HIV, was first identified in France[12]. In the description of the AIDS epidemic there are three patterns.

Pattern I describes the pattern seen in industrialised countries such as the United States of America, Europe, Canada and Australia, where the majority of AIDS cases are in homosexual and bisexual men. In these countries many more men than women have been diagnosed with AIDS. However, more recently there has been a shift and most newly reported AIDS cases are now among injecting drug users (IDU). This has major implications for heterosexual transmission, and there is already evidence that the number of women and children with AIDS is increasing[13,14].

Pattern II is seen in Africa, the Caribbean and some countries of South America, where most people with AIDS have acquired their infection heterosexually. Approximately equal numbers of males and females are infected and paediatric infection is a major problem.

Pattern III countries are those where few AIDS cases have been diagnosed and where HIV infection is restricted to people who have had contact with Pattern I or II countries. Pattern III countries include Asia and the Middle East, although recently HIV infection among injecting drug users and prostitutes in some Asian countries has increased dramatically and is cause for serious concern[15,16].

These patterns provide a rough guide to the present situation, but the prevalence of AIDS and HIV infection in individual countries depends not only on the prevalence of infection in certain groups such as prostitutes and IDU, but also on the relative size of these groups in the general population.

Reporting of AIDS

In most countries newly diagnosed AIDS cases are reported centrally. In the USA this is to the Centers for Disease Control (CDC) in Atlanta, in the UK to the Communicable Diseases Surveillance Centre (CDSC) of the Public Health Laboratory Service, and the Communicable Diseases Unit in Scotland. The World Health Organisation (WHO) collates all reports of cases of AIDS world wide and has a collaborating centre in Paris which receives reports from the European region. It must be emphasised that AIDS will be under-diagnosed and under-reported, especially on a world wide basis.

By the end of February 1991, WHO had received reports of 334,215 cases of AIDS from 179 countries. In the USA, by February 1991, 164,129 people had been reported with AIDS and in Europe by the end of February 1991 there were 47,481 cases. The 83,249 reports from Africa are almost certainly a gross underestimate of the true situation since many cases are likely to remain undiagnosed, particularly in areas where diagnostic facilities are lacking and mechanisms for reporting are minimal. The majority of African cases are from Uganda, Zaire, Kenya and Tanzania[17].

In contrast to Africa, where equal proportions of men and women are infected, in the USA and Europe only approximately 10 per cent of the total number of AIDS cases are women. In Europe there were 5948 reported AIDS cases in women by the end of December 1990 (of whom 182 were from the UK). The majority of these women were of childbearing age and 56 per cent were IDU[18]. The increasing numbers of women with AIDS has been parallelled by an increasing number of children with AIDS[17]. By the end of December 1990, 2120 children had been reported with AIDS in Europe. Although a substantial number of these children had acquired infection through infected blood or blood products, the number of new HIV infections in this category is not likely to increase significantly. However, the inclusion of 1094 cases from Romania highlights the need for vigilance in the use of needles, syringes and the testing of blood. The most important mode of infection for the 2120 children with AIDS was mother-to-child transmission. Figures 1.1 and 1.2 show the mode of acquisition of infection for the mothers of these children with or without the 1094 cases from Romania. France (271), Spain (247) and Italy (204) reported the largest number of cases. This is due to the high prevalence of HIV infection in the injecting drug user population in Italy and Spain, and the increasing heterosexual transmission of HIV in France. In the UK, there were 58 reports of children with AIDS, 36 of whom were due to mother-to-child transmission. (For the number of children with haemophilia and HIV infection in the UK see Chapter 4, Part 1.)

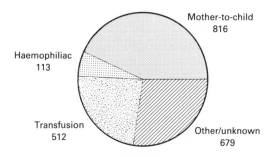

Fig. 1.1 Paediatric AIDS in Europe including Romania. Reproduced from *WHO Quarterly Report no. 28*, Geneva, WHO.

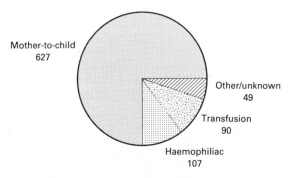

Fig. 1.2 Paediatric AIDS in Europe excluding Romania. Reproduced from *WHO Quarterly Report no. 28*, Geneva, WHO.

HIV infection

AIDS is a syndrome of symptoms and signs resulting from the damage to the immune system caused by HIV. It represents the end-stage of HIV infection and the incubation time from infection to development of symptoms can be long (see Chapter 3). Studies of groups of individuals in whom the time of infection was known suggest that the median time from infection to AIDS is about 10 years[19,20,21,22]. This means that although a few people develop AIDS soon after they have become infected with HIV, many will remain asymptomatic for prolonged periods. It should be emphasised that these people can pass on the infection even if they themselves may not be aware that they are infected. In terms of the description of the epidemic it is therefore more appropriate to have knowledge of the prevalence of HIV in a population and the characteristics of those with infection, rather than of the number of cases of people with AIDS. However, in the absence of mandatory population screening this is not possible, and current knowledge is based on those individuals who come forward to be tested. This is likely to be biased towards those who are in contact with medical services, for example, pregnant women, those with symptoms, injecting drug users (IDU) and attenders of sexually transmitted diseases clinics. Reports from the USA suggest that selective testing is inefficient in identifying seropositive pregnant women because some women do not know that they are at risk whilst others do not wish to disclose this[23,24].

In the UK information on HIV infection is mainly derived from laboratory reports[25]. By the end of December 1990, 1,553 HIV-seropositive females had been reported: 10 per cent of all HIV-positive people in England, Wales and Northern Ireland and 25 per cent of those in Scotland. The higher proportion of HIV-positive women in Scotland reflects the high prevalence of infection in the IDU population and demonstrates how even within the UK the pattern of infection can vary. In the UK by the end of December 1990 there had been 423 reports of HIV antibody-positive children of whom 198 were born to infected mothers[25]. As a substantial proportion of these children were under one year of age and maternal antibody may persist in the child for up to 18 months, it is not possible to determine without follow-up how many of these children are infected.

Unlinked anonymous testing of blood taken for other purposes should provide a better estimate of prevalence in the general population[26], although even this is limited to those people who need to have their blood taken. Such studies are now in progress. Table 1.1 gives the prevalence of HIV infection in antenatal women derived from blood taken routinely from newborns[27,28,29,30], or from women in the antenatal period[31].

Current policy for pre-natal testing in the UK concentrates on individuals at high risk for acquisition of HIV infection[5]. *No* screening programme should be embarked upon without adequate resources for pre- and post-test counselling. The depth and extent of pre-test HIV counselling will vary with the circumstances; additional counselling and continued support is essential for

Table 1.1   Prevalence per 1000 of HIV infection in pregnant women

London, newborns	0.24
Italy, newborns	1.30
Massachusetts, USA, newborns	2.10
New York, newborns	6.60
Sweden, antenatal	0.13

any individual for whom a positive result is obtained.

New initiatives have been set up through the Royal College of Obstetricians and Gynaecologists[32] and the British Paediatric Surveillance Unit[33] to collect confidential and anonymous information on pregnancies complicated by HIV infection and to follow-up infants who are seropositive so that their infection status can be determined.

Pregnancy and HIV infection

It has been suggested that pregnancy accelerates the course of HIV infection in an infected woman[34]. As a result women have been advised to have a termination of pregnancy to protect their own health. However, this finding has not been substantiated in more recent prospective studies comparing pregnant and non-pregnant infected IDUs[35]. Further information is needed to clarify this issue, especially for symptomatic women.

Studies in Africa[36,37] have shown an increase in adverse pregnancy outcomes in seropositive women; infants of seropositive mothers were more likely to be premature and of low birthweight and to have a higher neonatal mortality rate than infants of seronegative mothers. There was no difference in the rate of abortion or stillbirth. These findings have not been confirmed by others and in prospective studies where most women are asymptomatic, HIV infection has not been associated with an increased risk of adverse pregnancy outcome[38,39].

In a study in New York of 39 seropositive and 58 seronegative pregnant women enrolled in a methadone programme, there was no difference in the frequency of spontaneous or elective abortions, ectopic pregnancies, preterm deliveries, stillbirths or low birthweight, nor was there a difference between the groups in antenatal, intrapartum or perinatal complications[38]. In European prospective studies, birthweight was related to maternal drug use during pregnancy rather than to HIV infection in the child; those mothers who injected drugs during pregnancy had smaller babies[40,41]. The adverse outcome found in the study by Ryder *et al.*[36] could reflect the higher prevalence of illness in the mothers as well as other adverse AIDS-related family factors which would be likely to affect the nurture and care given to the infant. Although low birthweight has been associated with advanced HIV disease, it is not clear whether this is due to the direct effect of HIV infection in pregnancy or to a general effect of illness in the mother.

Mother-to-child transmission of HIV

Vertical transmission from mother to child may occur before, during or shortly after birth, but in view of the difficulty in making an early diagnosis the relative contribution of each of these routes remains unknown. There is clear evidence that transmission of HIV infection can occur before birth: virus has been found in fetal tissue from as early as 15 weeks gestation[42] and virus may be present in umbilical cord blood[36]. The very early onset of AIDS in some children is also suggestive of intrauterine infection[40,41]. Since HIV may be present in cervical secretions and there is the added risk of exchange of blood between mother and child during the delivery, transmission of HIV during birth remains a possibility (in analogy with Hepatitis B). Post-natal transmission of HIV infection through the ingestion of breastmilk has been described in several case reports where a breastfeeding mother acquired the infection shortly after birth through a blood transfusion and where the child was subsequently found to be infected[43]. The virus has also been found in breastmilk[44]. However, in situations where the mother acquires infection after delivery, she is likely to be more infectious in view of the circulation of free virus in the absence of antibodies. The added risk of transmission of HIV infection through breastfeeding from a woman who was already HIV antibody positive during pregnancy is unknown, but is thought to be small and has not been demonstrated in prospective studies. Nevertheless in many countries, the government guidelines state that where safe alternatives are available, HIV-positive mothers should be discouraged from breastfeeding. WHO guidelines explicitly encourage breastfeeding in developing countries, irrespective of HIV infection status. (See also Chapters 6 and 7.)

Difficulty of early diagnosis

The presence of HIV antibodies in a child whose mother is not infected, such as a child who has received contaminated blood products, is indicative of infection. However, for children born to HIV-seropositive mothers, diagnosis poses a problem (see also Chapter 2). Maternal HIV antibody crosses the placenta, so that the presence of HIV antibodies in a young child may merely indicate maternal infection and maternal antibodies may persist well into the second year of life. The diagnosis of HIV infection in a child born to an HIV-positive woman, based on the presence of HIV antibodies, will therefore have to wait until the child is 18 months of age. Although HIV infection can also be diagnosed by the detection of virus or viral antigen, these tests are expensive, can only be performed in specialised laboratories and are not available for routine diagnostic purposes. Also, failure to detect virus does not exclude infection and detection of antigen is less useful because it reflects disease progression. The recently described polymerase chain reaction method of diagnosis of HIV infection amplifies the viral genetic material so that minute quantities of virus can be detected (see Chapter 2). This method looks encouraging but is still at the research stage and will need to be carefully evaluated before it can be applied more widely.

The difficulty of early diagnosis poses a problem for parents, the child's carers and clinicians; it complicates decisions about treatment and poses particular difficulties for adoption and fostering. (See also Chapter 9.)

Rates of vertical transmission

Estimates of rates of vertical transmission vary widely. Initially estimates were based on studies of small and selected groups of children. The bias towards children or mothers with symptoms or mothers who already had an infected child is likely to have overestimated the risk of transmission[45,46]. More recently results have become available from prospective studies where children born to HIV antibody-positive women are identified before or at birth and followed up until their infection status can be determined. The estimated rates of vertical transmission from these studies vary from 13 to 39 per cent[36,37,40,41,59]. Differences in estimated rates of transmission can be accounted for in part by differences in methodology and samples studied. The higher rates found in Africa could be due to the fact that more of the mothers are symptomatic and therefore more infectious. Different strains of the virus could also possibly explain some of the variation of rates of vertical transmission. However, many questions remain and further research is necessary.

It is not known why some children born to HIV antibody-positive mothers are infected whereas others are not. As with other infections, even in a single pregnancy only one twin may be infected[47,48]. It has been suggested that the mother's clinical status during pregnancy influences the likelihood of infection in her child, with symptomatic mothers more likely to transmit the infection to the child[36]. However, although this is plausible it remains circumstantial and firm evidence is lacking. In the European Collaborative Study[41] the mother's clinical status was not related to the child's HIV infection. Mode of delivery could be a risk factor in the transmission of HIV infection from mother to child, with a vaginal delivery increasing the likelihood of transmission. However, evidence from prospective studies to date[40,41] shows no difference in rate of transmission according to mode of delivery and there is no evidence that delivery by caesarean section would reduce the risk. In the European Collaborative Study of children born to HIV-positive mothers, despite the relatively large number of children in the study, it is still not possible to give reliable risk estimates for these variables due to the small numbers of children in each category. Recently the presence of certain antibodies has been described[49] which may protect the child against transmission of HIV. However, these results are preliminary and need to be substantiated.

Classification of paediatric HIV infection

The CDC classification for paediatric HIV infection[50] is based on clinical manifestations and laboratory findings in relation to age (Table 1.2). (See also Chapter 3.) Children born to HIV-seropositive mothers and who are antibody positive but aged less than 15 months, are of indeterminate infection status. In the European Collaborative Study, 18 months of age was considered to be more appropriate, as a substantial number of children become antibody negative between 15 and 18 months of age. Class P1 refers to children who are asymptomatic but known to be infected with or without immunological abnormalities, and class P2 refers to symptomatic children. The various

Table 1.2 CDC classification of paediatric HIV infection

Class P-0	Indeterminate infection
Class P-1	Asymptomatic infection
	A Normal immune function
	B Abnormal immune function
	C Immune function not tested
Class P-2	Symptomatic infection
	A Non-specific findings
	B Progressive neurological disease
	C Lymphoid interstitial pneumonitis
	D Secondary infectious disease
	E Secondary cancers
	F Other diseases possibly caused by HIV infection

Reproduced from Centers for Disease Control (1987). *MMWR*, **36(15)**, 225–36.

categories within class P2 indicate the symptomatology. This classification is likely to be revised as further information on the natural history becomes available.

Where laboratory information cannot be obtained, the WHO clinical definition of AIDS[51] is useful in identifying children with AIDS, but its sensitivity and specificity are not high and vary according to the prevalence of conditions in the population, such as malaria[52]. (See Table 1.3.)

There is a paucity of information on the natural history of HIV infection in children, largely due to the difficulty of regular and long term clinical and laboratory follow-up from birth. The clinical presentation of HIV infection is often non-specific and may involve a wide spectrum of clinical disease, including persistent generalised lymphadenopathy, persistent hepatomegaly, persistent splenomegaly, diarrhoea, fever unexplained by other causes, failure to thrive and parotitis. Other more serious manifestations include persistent oral *Candida*, lymphoid interstitial pneumonitis, progressive encephalopathy and opportunistic infections. The prognosis is variable and may depend on the presenting symptoms and age at diagnosis. Some children present with symptoms early in the first year of life with rapid progression to AIDS, and the mortality in this group is high. Some children may be severely debilitated for a long period of time, whereas others may have symptoms which are compatible with a normal life and school attendance. Only a small proportion of infected children remain symptom free beyond the age of two years. (See also Chapter 3.)

The incubation period of HIV infection from initial exposure to the onset of AIDS is variable and in vertically infected infants may well be bimodal[40,41,53]. Estimates based on children reported with AIDS in New York gave a short median incubation period of 4·1 months and a longer one of 6·1 years, resulting in an overall median incubation period of 4·8 years[53]. In most of the prospective studies follow-up has not yet been long enough to establish a bimodal distribution, although the majority of cases of AIDS reported have been in the first year of life. Some infected children develop AIDS at a very early age, but others may live for years without developing AIDS[40,41,54] even if they have HIV-related symptoms or signs.

In a recent paper Scott *et al.*[54] described the natural history of a group of HIV-infected children most of whom were first identified because of symptomatic disease. The median age of presentation of symptoms was eight

Table 1.3 WHO (1985) clinical case definition for paediatric AIDS. Paediatric AIDS is suspected in an infant or child presenting with at least two major signs plus at least two minor signs, in the absence of known causes of immunosuppression

Major signs	weight loss or abnormally slow growth
	chronic diarrhoea > 1 month
	prolonged fever > 1 month
	asthenia > 1 month
Minor signs	generalised lymphadenopathy
	oropharyngeal candidiasis
	repeated common infections
	persistent cough
	generalised dermatitis
	confirmed maternal HIV infection

Reproduced from WHO (1985). Workshop on AIDS in Central Africa, Bangui, Central African Republic. WHO/CDS/SIDA/85.1. Geneva, WHO.

months and 21 per cent presented after two years. The most common manifestations were lymphoid interstitial pneumonitis (17%), encephalopathy (12%), recurrent bacterial infections (10%) and *Candida* oesophagitis (8%). Mortality was high in the first year of life and the long term survival was low. In view of the short interval between birth and the onset of symptoms they emphasised the need for early diagnosis of infection so that prophylactic or antiviral treatment could be given before progression of disease.

It should always be borne in mind that children born to HIV-positive women may be socially disadvantaged and some of the more non-specific symptoms or signs may reflect social conditions rather than HIV infection *per se*[55]. The dysmorphic syndrome described in children born to HIV antibody-positive mothers[56] has not been confirmed by others, and it has been suggested that the syndrome was caused by drug use in pregnancy[40,41,57,58].

A team approach to the management of HIV infection is essential and both the children and their mothers (indeed the whole family) need support. (See also Chapters 8, 9 and 11.) Many mothers will require home visits by experienced nurses and/or social workers and it is important that a named paediatrician is given overall responsibility for the infant's follow-up, diagnosis of infection and clinical management (see Chapter 3). Illness in the mother may have consequences for the care of the child in the short and long term, irrespective of the infection status of the child. In addition to HIV infection, families may have to face other major problems such as those relating to finance, housing, injecting drug use, relationships and racial prejudice. The need to educate health professionals and the public about HIV infection and the routes by which it is acquired and how it can be prevented is essential and must be carried out on a continuing basis if these families are to be helped and not ostracised from society.

References

1. Senturia, Y. D., Peckham, C. S. (1987). Pre-school immunisation: the importance of achieving adequate uptake. *Children and Society*, **3**, 198–209.
2. Rogers, M. F., White, C. R., Sanders, R. *et al.* (1990). Lack of transmission of human immunodeficiency virus from infected children to their household contacts. *Pediatrics*, **85**, 210–14.
3. Reed Shirley, L., Ross, S. (1989). Risk of transmission of human immunodeficiency virus by bite of an infected toddler. *J. Pediatrics*, **114(3)**, 425–7.
4. Centers for Disease Control (1988). Update: Universal precautions for prevention of transmission of human immunodeficiency virus, hepatitis B virus and other blood-borne pathogens in health-care settings. *Morbidity and Mortality Weekly Report*, **37**, 377–88.
5. Royal College of Obstetricians and Gynaecologists (1987). *Report of the RCOG Sub-committee on Problems Associated with AIDS in Relation to Obstetrics and Gynaecology*. RCOG, London.
6. Department of Health (1990a). *HIV – The Causative Agent of AIDS and Related Conditions*. HMSO, London.
7. Department of Health (1990b). *Guidance for Clinical Health Care Workers: Protection Against Infection with HIV and Hepatitis Viruses*. HMSO, London.
8. WHO Collaborating Centre On AIDS (1989). AIDS surveillance in Europe. *WHO Quarterly Report no. 22*, 18–19.
9. Cameron, D. W., Simonsen, J. N., D'Costa, L. J. *et al.* (1989). Female to male transmission of human immunodeficiency virus type 1: Risk factors for seroconversion in men. *Lancet*, **ii**, 403–7.

10. Johnson, A. M., Laga, M. (1988). Heterosexual transmission of HIV. *AIDS*, **2(1)**, S49–56.
11. Rubinstein, A., Sicklick, M., Gupta, A. (1983). Acquired immunodeficiency with reversed T4/T8 ratio in infants born to promiscuous and drug-addicted mothers. *Journal of the American Medical Association*, **249**, 2350–6.
12. Vilmer, E., Fischer, A., Griscelli, C. (1984). Possible transmission of human lymphotropic retrovirus (LAV) from mother to infant with AIDS. *Lancet*, **2**, 229–30.
13. Centers for Disease Control (1990). Update: Acquired Immunodeficiency Syndrome – United States, 1989. *Morbidity and Mortality Weekly Report*, **39**, 81–6.
14. World Health Organisation (1990). Acquired Immunodeficiency Syndrome in 1989. *Weekly Epidemiological Record*, **16**, 117–22.
15. Smith, D. G. (1990). Thailand: AIDS crisis looms. *Lancet*, **335**, **i**, 781–2.
16. Gelmon, K. (1990). AIDS, San Francisco. *Lancet*, **i**, 1581–2.
17. World Health Organisation (1991). AIDS statistics. *AIDS*, **5(4)**, 471–4.
18. WHO Collaborating Centre On Aids (1990). *AIDS Surveillance in Europe.* WHO Quarterly Report no. 28, 31 December. WHO, Paris.
19. Goedert, J. J., Kessler, C. M., Aledort, L. M. *et al.* (1989a). A prospective study of human immunodeficiency virus type 1 infection and the development of AIDS in subjects with haemophilia. *New England Journal of Medicine*, **321(17)**, 1141–8.
20. Schechter, M. T., Craib, K. J. P., Le, T. N. *et al.* (1989). Progression to AIDS and predictors of AIDS in seroprevalent and seroincident cohorts of homosexual men. *AIDS*, **3(6)**, 347–54.
21. Moss, A. R., Bacchetti, P., Osmond, D. *et al.* (1988). Seropositivity for HIV and the development of AIDS or AIDS related condition: three year follow-up of the San Francisco General Hospital cohort. *British Medical Journal*, **296**, 745–50.
22. Anderson, R. M., Medley, G. F. (1988). Epidemiology of HIV infection and AIDS: incubation and infectious periods, survival and vertical transmission. *AIDS*, **2(1)**, 57–64.
23. Minkoff, H. L., Holman, S., Beller, E. *et al.* (1988). Routinely offered prenatal HIV testing (correspondence). *New England Journal of Medicine*, **319**, 1018.
24. Krasinski, K., Borrowsky, W., Bebenroth, D., Moore, T. (1988). Failure of voluntary testing for human immunodeficiency virus to identify infected parturient women in a high-risk population (correspondence). *New England Journal of Medicine*, **318**, 185.
25. PHLS Communicable Disease Surveillance Centre (1991). Human immunodeficiency virus type 1 (HIV-1) antibody reports: United Kingdom: weeks 84/45–90/52. Acquired immune deficiency syndrome: United Kingdom: 1982– December 1990. *Communicable Disease Report*, **91/3**, 13–14.
26. Gill, O. N., Adler, M. W., Day, N. E. (1989). Monitoring the prevalence of HIV. *British Medical Journal*, **299**, 1295–8.
27. Ippolito, G., Stegagno, M., Costa, F. *et al.* (1989). Detection of anti-HIV antibodies in newborns: a blind serosurvey in 92 Italian hospitals [abstract]. In: *Les Implications du SIDA Pour le Mere et L'enfant*, p. 141.
28. Peckham, C. S., Tedder, R. S., Briggs, M. *et al.* (1990). Prevalence of maternal HIV infection based on unlinked anonymous testing of newborn babies. *Lancet*, **i**, 516–19.
29. Hoff, R., Berardi, V. P., Weiblen, B. J. *et al.* (1988). Seroprevalence of human immunodeficiency virus among childbearing women. *New England Journal of Medicine*, **318**, 525–30.
30. Novick, L. F., Berns, D., Stricof, R. *et al.* (1989). HIV seroprevalence in newborns in New York State. *Journal of the American Medical Association*, **261**, 1745–50.
31. Bohlin, A., Anzen, B., Arneborn, M. *et al.* (1989). HIV infection in pregnant women and perinatal transmission in Sweden [Abstract]. In: *V International Conference on AIDS. The Scientific and Social Challenge*, Montreal, June 4–9, p. 65.
32. Davison, C. F., Ades, A. E., Hudson, C. N., Peckham, C. S. (1989). Antenatal

testing for Human Immunodeficiency Virus. *Lancet*, **ii**, 1442–4.
33. Hall, S. M., Glickman, M. (1990). Report from the British Paediatric Surveillance Unit. *Archives of Disease in Childhood*, **65**, 807–9.
34. Scott, G. B., Fischl, M. A., Klimas, N. *et al*. (1985). Mothers of infants with the acquired immunodeficiency syndrome: Evidence for both symptomatic and asymptomatic carriers. *Journal of the American Medical Association*, **253**, 363–6.
35. Schoenbaum, E. E., Davenny, K., Selwyn, P. A. (1988). The impact of pregnancy on HIV-related disease. In: *AIDS and Obstetrics and Gynaecology*, Hudson, C. N. and Sharp, F., eds., Royal College of Obstetricians and Gynaecologists, London, pp. 65–75.
36. Ryder, R. W., Nsa, W., Hassig, S. E. *et al*. (1989). Perinatal transmission of the human immunodeficiency virus type 1 to infants of seropositive women in Zaire. *New England Journal of Medicine*, **320**, 1637–42.
37. Hira, S. K., Kamanga, J., Bhat, G. J. *et al*. (1989). Perinatal transmission of HIV-1 in Zambia. *British Medical Journal*, **299**, 1250–2.
38. Selwyn, P. A., Schoenbaum, E. E., Davenny, K. *et al*. (1989). Prospective study of human immunodeficiency virus infection and pregnancy outcomes in intravenous drug users. *Journal of the American Medical Association*, **261**, 1289–94.
39. Johnstone, F. D., MacCallum, L., Brettle, R. *et al*. (1988). Does infection with HIV affect the outcome of pregnancy? *British Medical Journal*, **296**, 467.
40. Blanche, S., Rouzioux, C., Guihard Moscato, M.-L. *et al*. (1989). A prospective study of infants born to women seropositive for human immunodeficiency virus type 1. *New England Journal of Medicine*, **320**, 1643–8.
41. European Collaborative Study (1988). Mother-to-child transmission of HIV infection. *Lancet*, **ii**, 1039–42.
42. Sprecher, S., Soumerknoff, G., Puissant, F., Degueldre, M. (1986). Vertical transmission of HIV in 15 week fetus. *Lancet*, **ii**, 288–9.
43. Oxtoby, M. J. (1988). Human immunodeficiency virus and other viruses in human milk; placing the issues in broader perspective. *Pediatric Infectious Diseases Journal*, **7**, 825–35.
44. Thiry, L., Spencer-Goldberger, S., Jonckheer, T. (1985). Isolation of AIDS virus from cell-free breast milk of three healthy virus carriers. *Lancet*, **ii**, 891–2.
45. Scott, G. B., Buck, B. E., Leterman, J. G. (1984). Acquired immunodeficiency syndrome in infants. *New England Journal of Medicine*, **310**, 76–81.
46. Friedland, G. H., Klein, R. S. (1987). Transmission of the human immunodeficiency virus. *New England Journal of Medicine*, **317**, 1125–35.
47. Couvreur, J. (1982). Congenital toxoplasmosis: the diagnosis colloque international sur l'immunologie dans la toxoplasmose. *Lyon Medical*, **248**, Suppl Nov 15, Fondation Marcel Merieux, Lyon, 125–32.
48. Menez-Bautista, R., Fikrig, S. M., Pahwa, S. (1986). Monozygotic twins discordant for the acquired immunodeficiency syndrome. *American Journal of Diseases of Children*, **140**, 678–9.
49. Goedert, J. J., Mendez, H., Drummond, J. E. *et al*. (1989b). Mother-to-infant transmission of human immunodeficiency virus type 1: association with prematurity or low anti-gp120. *Lancet*, **ii**, 1351–4.
50. Centers for Disease Control (1987). Classification system for Human Immunodeficiency Virus (HIV) infection in children under 13 years of age. *Morbidity and Mortality Weekly Report*, **15**, 225–36.
51. World Health Organisation (1985). Workshop on AIDS in Central Africa, Bangui, Central African Republic. *WHO/CDS/SIDA/85.1*.
52. Lepage, P., van de Perre, P., Dabis, F. *et al*. (1989). Evaluation and simplification of the World Health Organisation clinical case definition for paediatric AIDS. *AIDS*, **3**, 221–5.
53. Auger, I., Thomas, P., De Gruttola, V. *et al*. (1988). Incubation periods for paediatric AIDS patients. *Nature*, **336**, 575–7.
54. Scott, G. B. Hutto, C., Makuch, R. W. *et al*. (1989). Survival in children with perinatally acquired human immunodeficiency virus type 1 infection. *New England Journal of Medicine*, **321**, 1791–6.

55. European Collaborative Study (1990). Neurological signs in young children with HIV infection. *Pediatric Infectious Diseases Journal*, **9(6)**, 402–6.
56. Marion, R. W., Wiznia, A. A., Hutcheon, R. G., Rubinstein, A. (1987). Fetal AIDS syndrome score. *American Journal of Diseases of Children*, **141**, 429–31.
57. Qazi, Q. H., Sheik, T. M., Fikrig, S., Minkoff, H. (1988). Lack of evidence for craniofacial dysmorphism in perinatal human immunodeficiency infection. *Journal of Pediatrics*, **112**, 7–11.
58. Sheikh, T. M. (1987). Failure to confirm fetal AIDS syndrome (abstract). *Pediatric Notes*, **18(11)**, 70.
59. European Collaborative Study (1991). Children born to women with HIV-1 infection: natural history and risk of transmission. *Lancet*, **337**, 253–60.

2 Diagnosis of HIV infection

Sheila Burns and Jacqueline Mok

Consequences of infection with HIV

HIV is a member of the lentivirus sub-family of retroviruses. Characteristic properties of the sub-family include immunosuppression and a long incubation period. Although there are many retroviruses known in the animal and insect kingdom, HIV is one of only four viruses in the family which are as yet known to infect man (Table 2.1). (Information regarding the structure of HIV is given in Appendix 1, p. 22.)

Table 2.1 Retroviruses known to man

HTLVI	Human T cell lymphotrophic virus
	T cell leukaemia, tropical paresis
HTLVII	Human T cell lymphotropic virus
	Hairy cell leukaemia
HIV-1	Human Immunodeficiency Virus
	Immunosuppression, AIDS
HIV-2	Human Immunodeficiency Virus
	Immunosuppression, AIDS

Interference with host cell functions and fusion of infected cells to others leads to cell death. T4 helper lymphocytes, which have a central role in the immune systems defence against infection and also in the control of tumour formation by groups of cells, become depleted through this mechanism. The effect of HIV infection in an individual is the result of this progressive depletion of the T helper cells. HIV-infected lymphocytes are killed by other cells of the immune system, contributing to the decrease in numbers.

HIV-2 (see Appendix 1 on p. 25) has only infected a limited number of people so far. It has been associated with AIDS and has been transmitted from the mother to child (Table 2.2).

Table 2.2 Properties of HIV-2

Origin in West Africa
Distinct envelope glycoproteins
Closer homology to simian immunodeficiency virus
Unique *vpx* gene
Infects lymphocytes with CD4 molecule
Causes AIDS
May have longer incubation period than HIV-1
Transmission occurs from mother to child

Testing in clinical practice

Tests for HIV were originally developed to screen units of donated blood and to test selected and counselled persons at official clinics who were perceived to be at 'increased risk for HIV infection'. These tests were designed to detect antibody and various types of tests are available (Table 2.3). If samples are repeatedly reactive a confirmatory test is carried out. The tests are described more fully in Appendix 2 (pp. 25–9).

Table 2.3   Antibody tests for detecting HIV. (See also Appendix 2)

(a)   Enzyme-linked immunosorbent assay (ELISA)
   Whole viral lysate proteins
   Recombinant viral proteins
   Synthetic peptide proteins

(b)   Rapid immunoassays
   Particle agglutination tests
   Latex bead agglutination

(c)   Confirmatory testing
   Immunoblotting (Western blot)
   Immunofluorescence
   Radioprecipitation assay (RIPA)
   Virus neutralisation

Seroconversion

After initial infection with HIV the individual is infectious and antibodies to the virus develop within three months. During this three month period an individual can be infected without the development of antibodies that can be detected. This is sometimes referred to as the 'window period'. Acute primary infection is associated in some cases with clinical symptoms characterised by an acute glandular fever-type illness, with fever, sore throat, lymphadenopathy, fleeting macular rash and meningeal symptoms of headache, neck stiffness and mylagia. The mean duration of acute illness is 14 days[1]. During this illness virus can be cultured, HIV p24 antigen detected, and anti-HIV antibody develops. While the majority of children acquire infection by vertical transmission, post-natally acquired HIV may be associated with an acute HIV syndrome at the time of seroconversion. As yet little information is available in the literature.

Application of tests in infants

This is complicated by the presence of maternal HIV antibody which can cross the placenta from the mother to her infant. In most congenital virus infections, for example rubella, the level of passively transferred (IgG) antibody will be declining by three months and undetectable by 12 months. Maternal HIV IgG antibody can persist for over 15 months in an infant born to an HIV-infected mother. IgM class antibodies are not passively transferred, but manufactured by an infected infant. Detection of IgM class antibodies may be helpful. Detection of HIV virus or antigen by the methods described may also be helpful.

IgM and IgA class antibodies

In 'conventional' virus infections detection of IgM class antibodies which appear early after infection can be useful in diagnosing primary infection in an infant. This avoids the diagnostic difficulty of finding IgG antibodies which may have passively crossed the placenta from the mother (for example, rubella). Unfortunately, IgM cannot be reliably detected in infants infected with HIV. This is possibly because IgM is not produced by all such infants. The reasons why are not yet known. Whatever the reason IgM tests are not diagnostic. Detection of IgA HIV antibodies in infants at risk of HIV infection has been reported[2]. Preliminary studies indicate infants born to HIV-infected mothers have IgA HIV present in twice as many samples as IgM antibodies[3]. Detection of these IgA HIV antibodies may be an effective method of detecting HIV-infected infants before symptoms develop. These studies require further confirmation.

HIV antigen detection

Antigen detection involves incubating the patient's serum with HIV antibody bound to a solid support (see Appendix 2, p. 25). After incubation with an enzyme conjugated second antibody, a substrate is added to allow a chemical reaction to take place. The amount of antigen present can be calculated by measuring the intensity of colour which develops. This test can be made quantitative by the addition of samples of known quantity of antigen and the level of antigen is expressed in picograms per millilitre. Not all infected patients are p24 antigen positive in the early stages. The test detects free antigen in the serum which can become bound to antibody and thus be undetectable. The antigen does, however, reappear or appear late in the course of HIV infection. Antigen may be detectable up to one year before the onset of AIDS and it can be a useful indicator of the stage of disease. In children it may have a role in the monitoring of the response to treatment, when declining or disappearing antigen indicates less virus replication and so less disease activity.

Virus culture

This continues to be the reference method of determining HIV infection in a child. It is a costly and complicated technique and needs to be performed in laboratories with special safety facilities because it is possible that high titres of virus are generated. One further drawback is the large amount of blood required from the child – 5 ml.

In the laboratory the sample is processed and the lymphocytes removed. These are then added to special lymphocyte cell lines which have been stimulated. During this 'co-culture' procedure the HIV multiplies. An alternative method of culture involves stimulation of the patients lymphocytes on their own. P24 antigen is then measured in the supernatant, or the enzyme

Table 2.4   Body fluids which can be cultured for HIV

Saliva	Amniotic fluid
Breastmilk	Semen
Tears	Vaginal secretions
Cerebrospinal fluid (CSF)	Blood
Peritoneal, pericardial, pleural fluid	Plasma

reverse transcriptase is assayed. It is also possible to look at the cultures by electron microscopy for virus particles. As well as blood, other tissues and body fluids can be cultured for HIV (Table 2.4). These include saliva, tears, breastmilk, cerebrospinal fluid, peritoneal and pericardial fluids, amniotic fluid, semen and vaginal secretions. HIV has been isolated by culture from fetal tissue as early as eight weeks gestation. Cultures are maintained for four weeks before they are considered negative. It is much more difficult to isolate HIV from tissues rather than blood. Finding HIV in a child is definite evidence of HIV infection.

Detection of virus DNA

HIV can remain in a latent form for long periods within the cells. Molecular biology techniques are now available which allow detection of small numbers of infected cells in an individual. Using a technique called the polymerase chain reaction (PCR), small DNA sequences can be detected in the cells and plasma of infected individuals. This is a multi-step repetitive process (Fig. 2.1).

Initially *primers*, which are short sequences of DNA, are chosen which are complimentary to known sequences of HIV. These bind to the separated

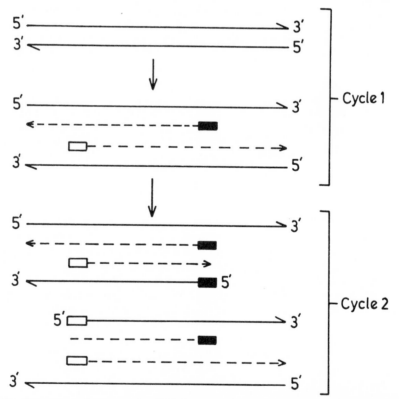

Fig. 2.1   Polymerase chain reaction (PCR). In *Cycle 1* the double strands of DNA are separated. Primers are introduced, which are short strands of bases with a mirror image to the existing HIV DNA single strands. These strands are enlarged using enzymes. In *Cycle 2* the four strands of DNA produced in cycle 1 are pulled apart and four similar primers added. The same procedure is repeated. This can continue for many cycles.

strands of HIV DNA and in the presence of a special enzyme called *taq* polymerase, extension of the sequences occurs. This process can be repeated for 30 or more cycles and the end result is the production of sufficient copies of the original DNA to be physically detectable. One single copy can be amplified one million times. This can be detected in several ways. Great care has to be taken to ensure the primers originally chosen are specific for viral HIV DNA and not cellular or other viral DNA. PCR has been shown to be an extremely sensitive technique. It has the advantage that it can detect latent as well as active infection. To date, preliminary studies have been very encouraging and once the problem of false positive results has been overcome, and the process automated, this method will assume a significant role in the diagnosis of HIV infection. It will be particularly useful in detecting HIV-infected children where maternal antibody is present.

Summary of testing in children

Diagnosis of HIV infection in infants is difficult. The presence of HIV antibodies in the infant at birth may be due to passively transferred maternal IgG. This maternal IgG can persist for up to 18 months and it is difficult to differentiate between maternal and infant antibody. Detection of serum antigen is helpful in some cases, but antigen is not likely to be present much before the onset of symptoms. Virus culture remains the reference method of diagnosing HIV-infected infants. PCR to detect virus sequence looks very promising as a way of early diagnosis in the asymptomatic stage.

Implications of testing

Specific guidelines have been recommended by the General Medical Council (1988) on testing for HIV infection. These have arisen, not because AIDS is different from other infections, but because of the recognised potential of serious social and financial consequences which follow because the patient has been tested and new information is known. In all circumstances doctors have to ensure that the patient's consent is obtained whenever investigative procedures are performed, in particular, those relating to HIV. This can be given implicitly, as when blood is obtained for multiple analyses, or explicitly when blood is tested specifically for a named condition. Good medical practice dictates that free exchange of information exists before any investigation or treatment is undertaken.

In the case of children, a particular difficulty arises because the child may have been infected by a parent, and testing the child implicitly tests the mother's HIV status. Where the parents withhold consent, the paediatrician must judge whether the child is competent to consent on his or her own behalf. If so, consent may be sought from the child. Should the child be unable or unfit to consent, the paediatrician must decide whether the interests of the child should override the wishes of the parent; and justify his or her action in testing without parental consent.

In paediatric practice, HIV testing arises in the following circumstances.

Diagnostic purposes

In the case of a child presenting with symptoms or signs which the paediatrician is expected to diagnose, this process is part of the consultation and consent is implied. It should be emphasised, however, that if HIV infection is strongly suspected parental consent must be specifically sought. The course of action to be taken in the event of non-cooperation from the parents has been outlined above.

Placement in care

Routine testing of all children received into care is *not* indicated as HIV transmission does not occur during casual household contact. (See also Chapters 1 and 9.) The Social Work Department, acting *in loco parentis*, may request testing, especially if risk activities are elicited from the parents. Due to the difficulties in interpreting serological results in the infant, testing often complicates rather than resolves the issue and is therefore not recommended.

Older children in care who are sexually active or who are injecting drug users present health care professionals with a dilemma. Consent to test for HIV should be discussed with the young person, unless there are specific contra-indications to this. The person named as *in loco parentis* will also be involved in this decision. It will be important for all concerned to understand the advantages and disadvantages of a test for HIV. Much consideration will have to be given to the youngster's reaction should the result be positive. This problem underlines the need for effective health education programmes.

Adoption

Adoption agencies must compile comprehensive medical reports on both the child and each birth parent. These should be available to all prospective adopters. Therefore, careful enquiry must be made into the mother's past history to elicit possible activities which may have put her at risk of HIV infection. She should then be counselled with a view to testing and, if HIV-positive, the status of her baby will still require to be determined. The adoptive parents may wish to pursue further investigations. Adoption agencies need to consider carefully the recruitment of adoptive parents as well as to ensure that expert advice is available to adoptive parents who wish to know more. There may be further pressure for HIV testing as the spread of HIV grows within the heterosexual population.

Sexually abused children

Although rare, the possibility exists that victims can be infected as a result of sexual abuse. Every effort should be made to discover the risk activities and the HIV status of the perpetrator. If necessary, blood can be taken and stored for HIV testing as part of the initial medical examinations and a repeat specimen sent to the laboratory six months later. The parents of the child should be offered careful counselling and the implications of a positive HIV result should be explained. They may not wish to have their child tested and their wishes should be respected. Storage of serum samples allows for retrospective testing should clinical indications arise. Most parents will agree to this.

Children with behavioural disorders

In schools for children with special needs there may be genuine reasons to identify children with specific disorders. These could include children who bite, who lack control of body secretions (such as urine and faeces) and those who have oozing skin lesions. They may be young, handicapped and disturbed. Such selected screening and assessment of a child whose personal conduct poses risks to others should always be considered on an individual basis, as each and every situation will require particular attention.

Where there is a child known to be at risk of HIV infection an experienced clinician will already be involved with the child, and advice should be sought. Parents, teachers and others closely involved with the child must also be included in the discussion.

Confidentiality

Difficulties concerning confidentiality are usually overcome if doctors are prepared to discuss fully with patients the implications of their diagnosis, the importance of continuing medical care and the need to secure the safety of others. In the case of children, a balance must be achieved between the assurance of proper care and the need to protect the family's privacy. Also, many agencies are involved in child care, with resultant demands of 'the right to know' the child's HIV status. (See also Chapters 5 and 9.)

Health care professionals

Many parents accept the need for the general practitioner and the health visitor to be informed of the diagnosis, without which they cannot be expected to provide adequate management and care. School medical officers have a unique role where children with signs and symptoms suggesting HIV infection may be referred by teaching staff. Prior knowledge of a child's HIV status will allow the school doctor to pay particular attention to deterioration in school performance or frequent absences, and so refer the child for a specialist opinion. (See also Chapter 8, Part 2.)

However, in some instances there has been marked reluctance on the part of some parents to allow various other health care professionals to become involved. This reluctance may be influenced by many factors, for example:

- the timing of such involvement. The parents may have been emotionally shocked due to a new diagnosis, or a recent bereavement.
- the trust and confidence that parents have already invested in a specific professional–patient relationship.
- the general knowledge of the stigma and anti-social attitudes that surround HIV and AIDS which reinforce the feelings of isolation. This may lead parents to feel they are vulnerable, out of control and victims of breached confidentiality.
- the parents need for continuity and consistency of medical and nursing care.

If parents refuse consent for other health care professionals to be informed of the child's, or parent's diagnosis, then the paediatrician has an obligation to maintain confidence. At all times, the family's request for privacy must be respected, except in the rare occasion when the doctor judges that a person *needs* to know, in which case the doctor must be able to justify his or her action. *All* health care professionals receiving such information are under the same obligation of confidentiality as the doctor who has principal responsibility for the patient's care. [There are many instances of adults with HIV-related illness being cared for in clinics of genito-urinary medicine and their children cared for by separate paediatric units. In such circumstances, the adults will be protected by the National Health Service (Venereal Diseases) Regulations 1974. There may be ethical and legal difficulties about sharing information between professional health care workers. It will always be important to gain consent, wherever possible, from the adult patient before relevant information can be exchanged. Ed.]

Other professionals

Educational establishments have been advised that it is safe for HIV-infected children to be integrated into mainstream schools without their identities being disclosed. Guidelines which advise on the handling of accidents which involve bleeding should therefore be adhered to, and education authorities must ensure that supplies of gloves and disinfectants are available to schools. Where the infected child has poor immune function, he or she is at risk of other infectious diseases and may require special educational provisions. Under these circumstances, many parents may consent to the disclosure of the child's diagnosis to the teaching staff. (See also Chapters 4, 8 and 12.)

Social work staff involved in child care include foster parents, day carers, community carers and staff in child care establishments. All should receive in-service training on HIV infection, with particular emphasis on the practical aspects of looking after infected children. The aim is to improve personal hygiene standards and to dispel the myths and stigma surrounding the disease. Regular handwashing, the covering of open lesions with waterproof plasters and the provision of gloves for dealing with significant bleeding are all that are required for *all* children. Emphasis on hygiene obviates the need to identify particular children who are HIV-infected, some of whom may not even be known to the medical profession! The same professional conduct applies to any member of staff who has been informed about the child and family's HIV status.

Alternative tests

There are several other markers of HIV infection. These include the absolute T helper cell (CD4) count, P24 antigen levels, B2 microglobulin levels and serum and urine neopterin levels. Use of these diagnostic tests in infected individuals can assist in assessing HIV activity. *It should be emphasised that if the HIV status is not known, any investigations related to HIV tests (including the alternatives) should only be carried out with full parental knowledge and consent wherever possible.*

Additional virological tests

Herpes viruses in AIDS

All six members of this group of viruses have a role in HIV-infected individuals (Table 2.5). Primary infection with these viruses usually occurs children who unlike adults, are more likely to experience reactivation of infection.

Herpes simplex type 1 (HSV 1)

Primary infection with HSV causes gingivostomatitis. A painful vesicular

Table 2.5 Herpes viruses in AIDS

Herpes simplex	Acute gingivostomatitis
Varicella	Disseminated chickenpox
Cytomegalovirus	Retinitis, adrenalitis
Epstein Barr virus	Lymphoma, hairy leukoplakia
Human Herpes virus 6	Disease acceleration

eruption occurs along the lip, tongue, pharynx or buccal mucosa. Necrotic ulcers can develop and fever and cervical lymphadenopathy are common. Affected infants have difficulty feeding. Antiviral therapy is safe and effective in treating severe infection. Diagnosis is made by culturing swabs from the nose and throat or electron microscopy of virus particles in vesicle fluid.

Varicella

Primary varicella (or chickenpox) infection in children with normal immune systems is usually mild. In children with lymphopenia (less than 500 lymphocytes per mm^3) infection is severe and prolonged (Table 2.6). Complications develop such as life threatening pneumonia and secondary bacterial infections. As with Herpes simplex, antiviral therapy in the form of acyclovir is available, and can be given with high titre varicella immunoglobulin (VZIG). (See Chapters 3 and 8, Part 2).

Table 2.6 Features of Varicella zoster in HIV-infected children

Life threatening
Can be recurrent
Tends to be chronic
Prolonged excretion of virus
Bacterial superinfection common
Responds to treatment

Cytomegalovirus (CMV)

Primary infection occurs in childhood or young adulthood in up to half the population depending on their social circumstances. In the immunocompromised child virus replication is prolonged and the virus is shed for long periods – for up to a year. All the herpes viruses share the property of becoming latent in the host and after primary infection the *cmv* genome remains latent in the cell. When the immune system is diseased for any reason, including HIV, the virus reactivates and begins to multiply. Serious infections of the eye, brain, lungs and adrenal glands can occur. This virus is more resistant to current antiviral drugs than Herpes simplex or varicella. Treatment is toxic and reserved for severe and life threatening disease.

Epstein-Barr virus (EBV)

Epstein-Barr virus (EBV) is another highly prevalent herpes virus which causes glandular fever in teenagers. This virus has a particular role in HIV-infected individuals. There is some evidence that EBV is involved in the immunological dysfunctions of HIV infection. EBV infects lymphocytes which are derived from the bone marrow (B lymphocytes). It is also known to infect similar cell types as HIV. Opportunist EBV infection produces three particular HIV-associated syndromes: lymphoid interstitial pneumonitis, lymphoma and oral hairy leukoplakia. Many children with AIDS have developed a chronic diffuse interstitial pneumonia. Parts of the EBV genome have been identified in biopsies from these children. Antibodies against the viral capsid antigen and early antigen are present in these children.

Human Herpes virus 6 (HHV6)

HHV6 is a recently recognised member of the Herpes family. It is the cause of exanthem subitum, one of the infective illnesses with rash usually experienced in childhood. Studies of serum from adults show more than half have antibodies to the virus. Cells in culture can be infected with both HIV and HHV6, and this causes acceleration of HIV turnover. Preliminary studies in man suggest this virus may have a role as a co-factor on disease.

Acknowledgements

Diagrams adapted from *Laboratory Diagnosis of Infection with the AIDS Virus*. Schochetman, G. Labmedica, April/May 1990, pp. 15–24.

References

1. Gaines, H., Sydow, M., Pearson, P., Lindbergh, P. (1987). Clinical picture of primary HIV infection presenting as a glandular fever-like illness. *British Medical Journal*, **297**, 1363–7.
2. Rakusan, T. A., Parrott, R. H. L., Sever, G. L. (1991). Limitations in the diagnosis in vertically acquired HIV infection. *Journal of Acquired Immune Deficiency Syndromes*, **4(2)**, 116–21.
3. Renom, G., Bouquety, J. C., Lanckist, C. (1990). HIV-specific IgA antibodies in tears of children with AIDS or at risk of AIDS. *Research in Virology*, **141**, 355–63.

Further reading

AIDS Guidance for Educational Establishments in Scotland. Scottish Education Department, 1987.
Children at School and Problems Related to AIDS. Department of Education and Science and Welsh Office. March 1986.
Clavell. (1989) *Virological and Clinical Features of HIV-2*. Current Topics in AIDS, Volume 2. John Wiley and Sons, Chichester.
General Medical Council. *HIV Infection and AIDS: The Ethical Considerations*. August 1988.
Mills, J. (1989) *Opportunist Infections in Patients with AIDS*. Marcel Dekker, New York.
Schoechetman, G. *Diagnosis of Infection with the AIDS Virus*. Labmedica. April/May 1990, pp. 15–24.

Appendix 1

Virus structure

The HIV genome contains group antigen (*gag*), polymerase (*pol*) and envelope (*env*) structural genes. These code for the proteins which are incorporated into the virus particle (Fig. 2.2).

HIV also contains three other genes which code for three regulatory proteins; regulator of viral protein (*rev*), transactivator (*tat*) and negative

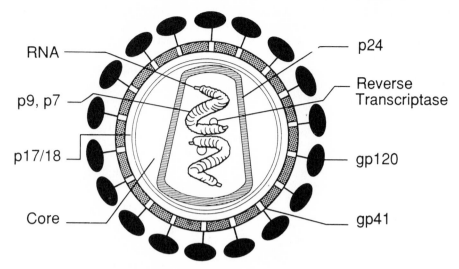

Fig. 2.2 Ultrastructure of HIV. The virus contains envelope proteins (gp41, gp120) and core proteins (p24, p18).

regulatory factor (*nef*). Three further protein products of three genes make up the virus. These are proteins thought to have a function in virus maturation and release of virus particles from the cell and are virion infectivity particle (*vif*) and viral proteins *u* and *r* (*vpu*, *vpr*). HIV-2 has the same number of structural genes, but has viral protein *x* (*vpx*) in place of *vpr*. The function of HIV proteins has been summarised in Table 2.7.

Table 2.7 Summary of HIV proteins

env gp160, gp120, gp41	envelope proteins
gag p55, p24, p17, p5, p9, p7	core proteins
pol p66, p51, p31	reverse transcriptase
tat p14	transactivator of virus
rev p19/p20	regulates expression
vif p23	infectivity factor
vpr	unknown
nef p27	reduces virus expression
vpu (HIV-1) p16	reduces virus release
vpx (HIV-2) p14	unknown

Infection of the cell takes place when the glycoprotein gp120, present in the outer envelope of the virus, interacts with the CD4 receptor on the surface of T helper lymphocytes (Fig. 2.3). Although no precise structure is known for the CD4 molecule as yet, a three dimensional structure has been proposed and it is known that there are at least two important binding sites (known as domains) on the gp120 molecule. Other cell types such as nerve cells and muscle cells do also bind HIV gp120 but the nature of these binding sites is not yet known. Once inside the cell the virus uncoats and releases its single strand of ribonucleic acid (RNA). The viral enzyme reverse transcriptase acts to produce DNA (called a provirus) which enters the cell nucleus and becomes incorporated into the host cell DNA. This reaction is catalysed by the virus enzyme integrase. Control of gene expression and so of virus replication depends on cell and virus coded factors.

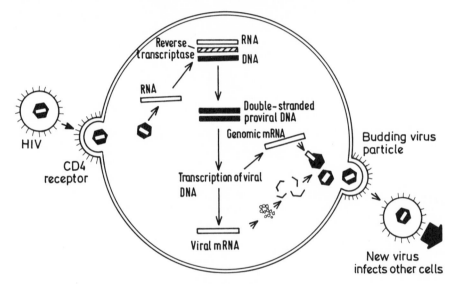

Fig. 2.3   Infection of a T helper lymphocyte with HIV.

Structural genes

The three main genes are *env*, *gag* and *pol*. *Env* codes for a glycoprotein gp160 which is then cleaved into two proteins, gp120, which forms the outer layer of the virus and gp41, which crosses the outer membrane and anchors the outer glycoprotein. The *gag* gene produces the proteins which form the core of the virus. These are p24, the protein which surrounds the RNA nucleus and p17 and p18 which are localised beneath the glycoproteins in the outer envelope (Fig. 2.2). *Pol* gene codes for the unique reverse transcriptase, the enzyme which is essential for the conversion of viral RNA into DNA which happens before the virus can begin to divide and replicate. Once the viral DNA is incorporated into the cell DNA it can remain latent or inactive for extended periods of time. Little is known about the factors which can maintain the virus latent for long periods.

The virus itself has three genes influencing viral expression and a complex interaction of these with cell factors may be responsible.

Regulatory genes

The *tat* gene is necessary for high levels of expression and it may do this by influencing nucleic acid binding. The second regulatory protein which is produced by the *rev* gene influences the export of messenger RNA from the nucleus to the cytoplasm where it is translated into protein. *Nef* is a 27 kilodalton protein associated with cell membranes and is a negative regulator of transcription and can hinder viral growth for example. It has been shown that strains of virus which do not contain the *nef* gene can grow to a higher titre in cell cultures. The later stages of HIV replication involve the assembly of the virus components into whole virus particles called virions. These are released from the cell by a process known as budding. The outer glycoprotein envelope of the virus will contain part of the cell membrane as a result of this budding process. The protein products of the genes are summarised in Table 2.7 (p. 23).

HIV-2

The overall organisation of the HIV-2 genome is very similar to that of HIV-1, with the major *gag*, *pol* and *env* genes. The unique HIV-2 gene, *vpx*, produces a protein which can be detected in the serum of infected patients but its function is unknown. Like HIV-1, HIV-2 also infects cells with the CD4 molecule on their surface. The envelope glycoproteins show some similarity but it is the core proteins of HIV-1 and HIV-2 which have the most in common.

HIV genome variability

HIV undergoes a genetic transmission from its RNA genome into a DNA provirus. This process, controlled by viral reverse transcriptase, is subject to error. Base substitution errors have been calculated to occur at a rate of $1:2000$ to $1:4000$ and this may account for the high mutability of HIV. As the virus replicates minor changes in the base composition lead to antigenic changes. For the genome of approximately 1000 bases, this means that the reverse transcription misincorporation is more than one base per replication cycle. As a result no two proviruses are identical. Changes in the HIV genome also seem to occur with time. Viruses isolated from asymptomatic patients are generally slow to grow in culture and can take three to four weeks to reach low titre. As the CD4 count drops and the patient becomes symptomatic, the virus isolated may grow rapidly reaching high titre within seven days.

Appendix 2

Antibody detected by enzyme-linked immunosorbent assay (EIA or ELISA)

(a)   Sandwich EIA or ELISA

Recombinant proteins are attached to either a polystyrene bead or a microtitre plate. Patients' serum is added and the bead or plate incubated. A second antibody to HIV (produced in an animal) which has an enzyme attached is added. This is further incubated with a chemical substrate and a colour reaction develops. Each test run contains known positive and negative samples as controls and the reaction is carefully monitored. A single serum or plasma which reacts is tested again (Fig. 2.4).

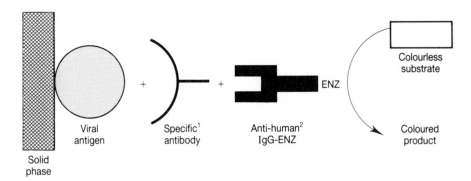

^{1} Patient serum
^{2} Horseradish peroxidase, Alkaline phosphatase, B-galactosidase, Glucose oxidase

Fig. 2.4   Enzyme-linked immunosorbent assay (ELISA).

(b)   Competitive EIA or ELISA

In this test the patient's sample is added to the plate or bead at the same time as a known antibody-positive control sample. These compete for binding to the HIV protein attached to the solid phase. The presence or absence of protein is again identified by a chemical reaction.

Confirmatory testing

In the Western blot assay, partially purified virus or a 'cocktail' of virus proteins are electrophoresed on a polyacrylamide gel to obtain separation of viral proteins. The bands obtained are then transferred on to a nitrocellulose membrane which can be cut into strips. When a test serum is incubated with the strip and an enzyme added, a coloured band will appear at the site of antigen antibody reaction (Fig. 2.5). A pattern of bands appears for each positive serum. Antibodies to the p24 core protein have been reported to appear earliest after infection and then decrease before the onset of clinical symptoms. Antibodies to the gp120 and gp41 envelope glycoproteins are detectable in nearly all HIV-infected patients, at all stages of infection. A Western blot is said to be positive when the bands detected include gp41 or gp120, p24 and p31 (polymerase) (Fig. 2.6). This strict interpretation allows maximum specificity. More recently, Western blots have been performed on urine from infected individuals and a similar pattern of bands were seen.

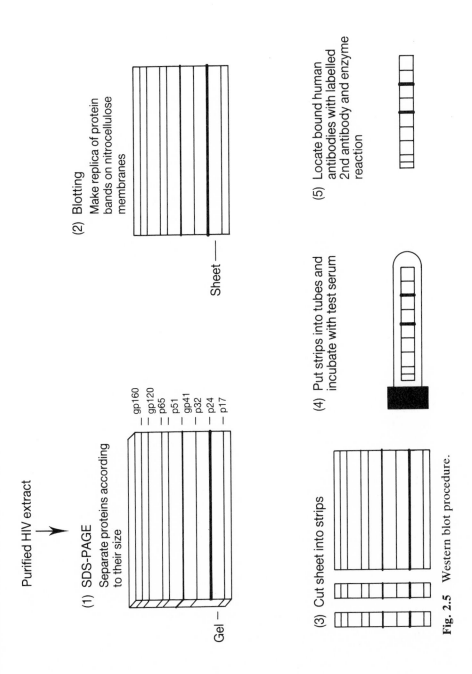

Purified HIV extract

(1) SDS-PAGE
Separate proteins according
to their size

gp160
gp120
p65
p51
gp41
p32
p24
p17

Gel —

(2) Blotting
Make replica of protein
bands on nitrocellulose
membranes

Sheet —

(3) Cut sheet into strips

(4) Put strips into tubes and
incubate with test serum

(5) Locate bound human
antibodies with labelled
2nd antibody and enzyme
reaction

Fig. 2.5   Western blot procedure.

Other methods of confirmation

Other methods of confirming initial positive reactions include the following:

(i)   Immunofluorescence

HIV-infected cells are inactivated and fixed to glass slides. Patients serum is then incubated with the infected cells and also with non-infected cells to act as a control. A further incubation then takes place with anti-human globulin

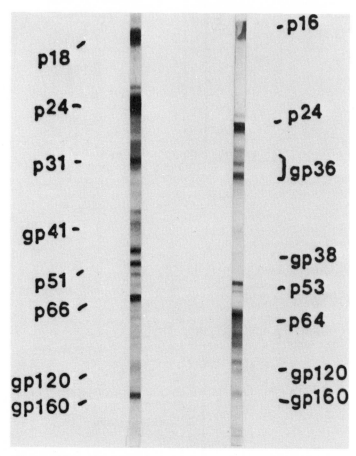

Fig. 2.6 Western blots of material from a patient infected with HIV. Bands are seen in the urine (left lane) and serum (right lane).

attached to a fluorescent dye. This will fluoresce in a specific manner when viewed by ultraviolet light.

(ii)   Radioprecipitation assay (RIPA)

This test involves feeding actively growing HIV-1-infected cells with media containing radiolabelled amino acids which become incorporated into viral proteins. Material obtained from these cells is reacted with patients' serum and radioactive complexes of HIV antigen/antibody are seen if HIV-specific antibodies are present in the patient's serum. This is a very sensitive test particularly for picking up envelope proteins, but because it is difficult to perform it is only performed in research laboratories.

(iii)   Neutralisation tests

Standard methods used for other viruses can be used for HIV.

3 The medical management of children with HIV disease

Jacqueline Mok

Introduction

As experience with HIV-infected children accumulates a wide spectrum of disease has emerged, from asymptomatic carriers through to children with mild illnesses and to those with classical signs and symptoms of AIDS. The incubation period is variable, ranging from approximately six months to several years, and probably depends on the mode of infection. For children under five years of age, the mean incubation period is 2.3 years; while for all children under 14 years it is 4.7 years.

The definition and classification of HIV infection in children has already been discussed in Chapter 1.

Babies with perinatal infection

Although HIV is transmitted *in utero*, neonates rarely present with AIDS. There may however be signs of congenital infection, for example, low birthweight, small-for-gestational-age, anaemia, jaundice, thrombocytopenia or hepatosplenomegaly. A dysmorphic syndrome has been described, although not widely documented[1]. (See Chapter 1.)

The initial presentation is usually outside the newborn period, between six to nine months of age. Infants may either present with the severe infantile form of HIV infection, with opportunistic infections, involvement of the central nervous system, as well as evidence of cellular and humoral immune deficiency. Some infants have the less progressive form of the disease, with non-specific signs and symptoms (Table 3.1).

The clinical course may vary, but with time there is progressive immune

Table 3.1 Non-specific signs and symptoms of HIV disease

Recurrent respiratory infections
Persistent lymphadenopathy
Recurrent diarrhoea
Frequent unexplained fever
Failure to thrive/weight loss
Oral thrush
Chronic dermatitis
Hepatosplenomegaly
Anaemia
Thrombocytopenia

Table 3.2   Recognised syndromes in paediatric HIV infection

Infectious complications	Bacterial
	Viral
	Fungal
	Opportunistic
Neurological disease	
Lymphoid hyperplasia syndrome	Polyglandular enlargement
	Lymphoid interstitial pneumonitis
Cutaneous manifestations	Infections
	Non-infectious presentations
Gastro-intestinal involvement	Diarrhoea
	Wasting
Haematological abnormalities	
Malignancies	Non-Hodgkin's lymphoma
	Polymorphic B cell lymphoproliferative disorder
Others	Nephropathy
	Cardiopathy
	Hepatitis

dysfunction accompanied by clinical deterioration. HIV is known to affect every organ of the body, and the recognised syndromes affecting children are listed in Table 3.2.

[The following symptomatology and clinical management also apply to children who have acquired HIV infection other than via the perinatal route. This includes those who received infected blood and blood products, and those infected through sexual contact or via infected needles and syringes, etc. Ed.]

Clinical manifestations of paediatric HIV infection

Infectious complications

Despite raised gammaglobulin levels recurrent bacterial infections are common. Clinical manifestations include respiratory sepsis (upper and lower respiratory tract infections), urinary infections skin and soft tissue infections, and meningitis. Infecting organisms include *Streptococcus pneumoniae*, *Haemophilus influenzae*, *Staphylococcus aureus* and Gram negative bacilli.

Common viral infections of the respiratory tract are also seen, together with more severe complications of childhood illnesses such as measles or chickenpox. With the deteriorating function of CD4 cells, opportunistic infections develop with organisms such as *Pneumocystis carinii*, *Candida albicans*, Varicella zoster virus and atypical mycobacteria.

Neurological disease

Direct involvement of the brain results in HIV encephalopathy. The frequency of central nervous system involvement has been reported to vary from 30–90 per cent of HIV-infected children[2,3,4]. The infected child presents with a delay or regression in developmental milestones and cognitive function. There is evidence of acquired microcephaly, progressive symmetrical motor deficits, abnormal tone and pathological reflexes. Seizures are infrequent. The cerebrospinal fluid may show normal biochemistry with normal cell counts, even in the presence of gross clinical signs. The presence of HIV antigen or a positive HIV culture from cerebrospinal fluid does not correlate with clinical findings. The course of HIV encephalopathy is progressive although the rate of progression varies between children.

Lymphoid hyperplasia syndrome

Polyglandular enlargement

Apart from persistent generalised enlargement of lymph nodes and hepatosplenomegaly, some children have recurrent attacks of parotitis with resultant parotid gland enlargement. Paratracheal or perihilar lymphadenopathy may be obvious on the chest X-ray. The lymphoid proliferation may affect the gastro-intestinal tract, epicardium, adrenal glands and skeletal muscle, and may predispose to B cell malignancies.

Lymphoid interstitial pneumonitis

Approximately 50 per cent of children meeting the criteria for AIDS have lymphoid interstitial pneumonitis (LIP), which has an insidious onset with a chronic non-productive cough and breathlessness on exertion. Characteristic diffuse reticulonodular shadowing is seen on the chest X-ray, which is non-responsive to antimicrobial therapy and worsens with time. Progressive disease leads to hypoxia and finger clubbing. Although a lung biopsy provides the definitive diagnosis, LIP can be presumed on the clinical and radiological findings[5].

Cutaneous manifestations

Infections

Persistent mucocutaneous candidiasis, occurring without concomitant antibiotic use and despite antifungal therapy, is often the first infection which leads to the diagnosis of HIV infection. Oral candidiasis may spread to involve the pharynx and oesophagus, and causes anorexia due to pain on swallowing.

Bacaterial skin infections are often due to *Staph. aureus*, with folliculitis, impetigo, cellulitis and skin abscesses being common presentations. With immune dysfunction, viral infections are also seen as disseminated molluscum contagiosum or mucocutaneous ulceration due to Herpes simplex viruses.

Non-infectious presentations

The majority of children with symptomatic HIV infection have non-infectious skin eruptions. Eczematous rashes, atopic dermatitis, and drug associated reactions have been described. Kaposi's sarcoma has been reported in about four per cent of children with AIDS, commonly amongst Negroid populations. Petechiae and purpura are the result of thrombocytopenia.

Gastrointestinal involvement

Diarrhoea

Diarrhoea can be caused by infectious agents such as salmonella species, *Cryptosporidium*, cytomegalovirus (CMV), and *Mycobacterium avium intracellulare* (MAI). The virus can also involve the gastrointestinal tract directly, leading to malabsorption. In such children, jejunal biopsy has shown evidence of non-specific villus atrophy. The resultant diarrhoea persists despite aggressive therapy.

Wasting

Infectious enterocolitis, malabsorption, oropharyngeal infections and anorexia all combine to result in malnutrition and cachexia in the terminal stages of HIV infection. In many developing countries, severe wasting in patients infected with HIV led to the description 'Slim disease'.

Haematological abnormalities

The blood film may reveal atypical lymphocytes at the time of seroconversion. Children with asymptomatic HIV disease often show normal lymphocyte counts, including T helper cell (CD4) numbers.

With disease progression, there is decline in CD4 numbers with absolute numbers remaining below 800 cells/mm^3. Neutropenia, especially low leucocyte counts, can exacerbate infectious complications and limit therapeutic options.

Thrombocytopenia is seen at various stages of HIV infection, and is the result of immune mechanisms. Bruising occurs when the platelet count drops to $<100 \times 10^9$/L, although sequential counts show that recovery in platelet numbers can occur with no specific treatment. Anaemia can be microcytic, due to iron deficiency, or macrocytic as a result of zidovudine therapy. In the presence of abnormal liver function tests, coagulation problems may occur.

Malignancies

Kaposi's sarcoma and the HIV-associated lymphomas are uncommon in children. In some children, a polyclonal, polymorphic B cell lymphoproliferative disorder has been described[6] where hyperplastic lymphoid nodules are seen in the lung and other organs. Long term studies are required to elucidate the relationship between this lymphoproliferative disorder and malignancies.

Other disorders

It is clear that all organs are involved in HIV infection, either directly or as a result of opportunistic infections. Hepatic involvement leads to elevated transaminase levels, and other infectious agents are seldom implicated. Biopsy and autopsy specimens show evidence of chronic active hepatitis.

Renal involvement results in proteinuria, with the nephrotic syndrome described in many HIV-infected children. Cardiovascular abnormalities seen include a congestive cardiopathy secondary to either LIP or nutritional deficiencies; and arteriopathy involving coronary arteries. Eye disease may be caused by opportunistic organisms, although perivasculitis of the retinal vessels has been described which was not attributable to known viral aetiologies.

Differential diagnosis

Children at risk

The non-specific early presentation of HIV infection has to be differentiated from other common paediatric problems, both congenital and acquired. The neonate with symptoms of drug withdrawal, thrombocytopenia and low birthweight should alert the necessity for a careful medical and social history from the mother. The following risk factors may need consideration:

- A current or previous history of injecting drug use or a sexual partner with the same.
- Multiple transfusions of blood and blood products at a time and place where blood was not screened for HIV.
- Sexual contact in an area where HIV infection is endemic.

These may make the diagnosis of maternal infection likely.

The mother should be counselled with a view to HIV testing prior to the neonate being tested. The presence of transplacentally acquired maternal HIV antibodies means that a positive test in the neonate is tantamount to surrogate testing of the mother. Absence of clinical disease in either parent does not rule out the possibility of congenital HIV infection, as infected parents are often initially asymptomatic, and the child may be the index case in the family. Confirmed maternal HIV infection is the most sensitive predictor of HIV disease in an infant presenting with suggestive symptomatology. (See also Chapter 2.)

The advent of donor screening and heat treatment of blood products have almost eliminated blood as a source of HIV infection. However, it is prudent to remember individuals who have received such treatment at a time before donors were routinely screened, and after HIV infection was first documented in that area.

Adolescents may place themselves at risk of infection through unprotected sexual intercourse and/or needle sharing drug use. Socially and emotionally deprived youngsters are more likely to be at risk. Anecdotal cases of HIV transmission due to child sexual abuse have been reported. Table 3.3 summarises risk factors for HIV infection in children.

Table 3.3 Children at risk of HIV infection

Maternal HIV infection
Risk activities elicited from either parent
Multiple transfusions between 1978–1985 (in countries where blood is now screened for HIV)
Treatment with blood products/multiple injections
Sexually active adolescent
Injecting drug use
Sexual abuse

Other immunodeficiencies

Primary and secondary causes of immunodeficiency which must be excluded include agammaglobulinaemia and hypogammaglobulinaemia, severe combined T and B cell immune deficiencies, severe malnutrition, congenital infections and therapy with immune-suppressive agents. HIV infection is usually easily distinguished from other immune deficiencies in childhood, with the demonstration of elevated serum immunoglobulin levels and T cell immunodeficiency, especially if epidemiological risk factors can be documented.

Investigations

Immune competence

A differential white count allows assessment of the total numbers of lymphocytes and neutrophils. Total T and B lymphocyte numbers can also be measured, along with T cell subsets. Although there are few published reports of the normal range of CD4 cells in the infant under two years of age, prospective studies of all infants born to HIV-infected women show that CD4 numbers are usually in excess of 2000 cells/mm^3 in uninfected infants.

Cell mediated immunity is assessed by mitogen and antigen stimulation of lymphocytes, although the usefulness of routine tests for T cell function is doubtful. Responses to mitogen stimulation could remain normal for prolonged periods in HIV-infected children.

Humoral immunity is usually abnormal before cell mediated immune dysfunction is seen. B cell abnormalities include polyclonal hypergammaglobulinaemia and subnormal responses to specific antigens. The hallmark of HIV infection in children is elevated levels of IgG, IgA and IgM, which often predate other laboratory abnormalities such as CD4 lymphopenia. Despite high IgG levels, deficiencies of subclasses of IgG have also been documented. In end stage disease, hypogammaglobulinaemia is usually seen, with severe immunocompromise.

Defective B cell function results in impaired antibody production, and suboptimal responses to primary as well as secondary courses of immunisation have been reported[7,8]. This is discussed further in the section on immunisation (see p. 42).

Markers of disease progression

The progressive activation and destruction of lymphocytes and macrophages lead to secretion of neopterin and B2 microglobulin. Several investigators have used these estimations in serum and urine specimens to assess the progression of HIV disease. Virological markers which are helpful are HIV antigen levels, the presence of cell free virus, as well as the *in vitro* growth characteristics of the virus.

Other laboratory investigations

The multisystem involvement of HIV disease means that a close working relationship has to exist between the clinician and laboratory workers. Radiological investigations which may be necessary are X-rays, ultrasound examination of the chest, abdomen and pelvis, and imaging techniques of the central nervous system. For the evaluation of infectious episodes, close liaison between bacteriological, virological and clinical personnel is essential so that proper specimens can be obtained, dispatched and processed without unnecessary delay. Biopsy specimens should be taken *after* prior consultation between physician, surgeon, pathologist and microbiologist.

Long term follow-up

Little is known of the risk of HIV transmission from an infected mother to her child, nor of the natural history of HIV infection in children. The route of infection may influence the course of the disease. The long-term outlook for infants born to infected mothers but who are themselves 'presumed uninfected', and infected children with asymptomatic or mild disease, needs to be determined. For these reasons, long term surveillance of children at risk of HIV infection is of great importance.

The setting up of one such clinic in Edinburgh[9] has allowed experience and expertise to be accumulated in one centre, and for professionals from various disciplines to work together. The follow-up procedure is outlined in Table 3.4. Ideally, contact should be established with the pregnant women in the antenatal period. The close monitoring of the infants' clinical and laboratory status means that early intervention can take place when evidence of HIV infection is identified. Surveillance should probably continue till the adolescent years in those children presumed uninfected until a definitive test is available. The practical aspects of this undertaking is, however, fraught with difficulties when the disease still carries a stigma.

Table 3.4   Follow-up procedure for children at risk of HIV infection (3–6 monthly intervals)

Review of	-growth
	-development
	-clinical evidence of HIV infection
Laboratory tests	
Haematological	-haemoglobin
	-white cell count and differential platelet count
Immunological	-IgG, IgA, IgM levels
	-T lymphocyte subsets
Virological	-HIV antibody, antigen
	-virus culture
Child care issues	
Immunisation	
Liaison, if necessary, with	-Physician
	-Social services
	-Education departments and establishments
	-Paramedical staff
	-Voluntary agencies/self help groups

[Bearing in mind the need for confidentiality where appropriate – Ed.]

Medical management of symptomatic children

The majority of children infected with HIV in the Western world have acquired the infection from their mother, many of whom may have needle sharing drug use implicated in either their partners' or their own lifestyle. Such families are usually from areas with multiple deprivation, where HIV infection is merely one more hardship to be borne. [There are also boys with haemophilia who have HIV infection (see Chapter 4). As time progresses, there will be more children infected with HIV born to parents without any previously known high risk factors. There are increasing numbers of children in the UK who have become infected whilst they or their parents lived in parts of the world where HIV infection is endemic. Ed.] There may be more than one infected member in the family and more than one generation affected. Complex challenges therefore face any professional dealing with the HIV-affected family. Therapeutic programmes are destined for failure if family, social and financial problems are not recognised, or if professionals choose to work in isolation.

Supportive and general care

Families need counselling to come to terms with the stresses and stigma produced by the diagnosis of HIV infection. The fear of social rejection may cause many families to withhold the diagnosis from close members, thus denying themselves support. Where the mother is infected guilt is mixed with denial, and offers of help may be refused. Some mothers focus on the child's symptoms and deny their own infection, and it is therefore important that infected parents receive counselling and medical care from adult physicians. Death or illness in the mother may mean that alternative care facilities have to be found for the child. (See Chapters 9 and 11.)

The current mainstay of therapy for most HIV-infected children is close monitoring of growth and development, and prompt intervention during infectious episodes. The collaboration of a dental hygienist and dentist is essential so that a healthy diet and regular dental hygiene can be instituted, thus avoiding periodontal disease and caries.

Nutrition

Regular measurements of weight, height and head circumference allow detection of signs of failure to thrive. Where the weight is static, or 'falls off', advice from a paediatric dietitian must be sought. Even in early disease, attention must be paid to the child's diet, as many families with inadequate incomes find it difficult to prepare nourishing diets for children. Initially, caloric supplementation may be sufficient to achieve optimal growth.

As with most chronic diseases, children can become anorexic. The child with oropharyngeal candidiasis will be even more reluctant to eat. Nasogastric or nasojejunal feeding may be necessary, and this can be done intermittently (overnight) or continuously. Where there is evidence of malabsorption, protracted diarrhoea or vomiting, total parenteral nutrition may be the only means of providing adequate calories and fluids. Indwelling catheters have been used for parenteral nutrition in HIV-infected children with no increase in infective episodes or catheter complications reported when compared to those seen in oncology patients. The introduction of indwelling catheters means that close monitoring is necessary, and with assistance from the home care team some families can cope with the child at home.

Intractable diarrhoea leads to severe weight loss, and may persist despite parenteral nutrition. Microbiological investigations and empirical therapy are usually unhelpful. The use of zidovudine (AZT) has been advocated on the basis that the diarrhoea results from direct HIV infection of the gut.

Infections

As opportunistic infections in HIV-infected children are usually a primary rather than a reactivated infection, the range of organisms seen in all infectious episodes will be described.

Bacterial infections

In spite of elevated serum immunoglobulin levels, HIV-infected children show clinical evidence of humoral deficiency and are prone to recurrent bacterial infections. Respiratory symptoms are common, and prompt treatment should be commenced with broad spectrum antibiotics until culture results and sensitivities are available. Regular bacteriological surveillance, with nose and throat swabs, may assist in the choice of antibiotic. Prophylaxis against bacterial infections can be used, with either cotrimoxazole or regular infusions of immunoglobulin. Both have been shown to result in a reduction in the number of infectious episodes. The results of a multicentre study comparing the efficacy of intravenous immunoglobulin therapy versus placebo are awaited. Infusions of immunoglobulin can be given at a dosage of 200–400 mg/kg, at 2–4 weekly intervals. Its routine use remains controversial.

An increase in the incidence of tuberculosis has been reported in individuals with HIV infection. Therapy is usually prolonged, and requires several anti-tuberculous agents. Disseminated infection with atypical mycobacteria occurs in terminally ill children, for which there is no effective therapy at present.

Viral infections

Few effective antiviral agents exist, which limits treatment options for viral infections. Those children receiving regular intravenous immunoglobulin infusions may be protected against infection with common viruses. A history of exposure to measles, chickenpox or shingles in an immune-compromised child should be taken seriously, and hyperimmune globulin should be administered. Varicella zoster infections have severe complications, so that all primary infections and Herpes zoster should be treated promptly with intravenous acyclovir. Chronic cutaneous lesions due to Varicella zoster or Herpes simplex viruses may require prolonged therapy with acyclovir.

Some children are asymptomatic carriers of cytomegalovirus (CMV). With immune dysfunction, disseminated infection involving the lungs, gastrointestinal tract and central nervous system occurs. CMV retinitis leads to acute onset of blindness, and ganciclovir has proven efficacy in adults, although relapses occur when therapy is discontinued. Toxic effects of the drug include anaemia and neutropenia.

Fungal infections

Candidiasis affecting the mouth and nappy area is the commonest fungal infection seen in HIV-infected children. Local treatment with nystatin or miconazole is often prolonged, with relapses seen on cessation of treatment. With oesophageal or systematic candidiasis, fluconazole or ketoconazole have been shown to be effective. Refractory cases will require amphotericin B, which causes gastro-intestinal upset.

Cryptococcal meningitis may lead to disseminated infection. Therapy involves a course of amphotericin B and flucytosine for six weeks, despite which relapses occur. Treatment is often poorly tolerated due to bone marrow suppression.

The commonest opportunistic pathogen in children with AIDS is *Pneumocystis carinii*. [The classification of this pathogen is a subject of current debate. Ed.] Onset of *Pneumocystis carinii* pneumonia (PCP) is usually rapid, with cough, fever and tachypnoea. Clinical and radiological findings may be minimal, but hypoxia is always present and merits oxygen therapy. Diagnostic difficulties arise owing to the difficulties in obtaining induced sputum specimens from young children, who may be too ill to tolerate broncho-alveolar lavage or lung biopsy. Recently, the use of monoclonal antibodies has allowed the rapid diagnosis of PCP from nasopharyngeal secretions[10]. Pending results, treatment is empirical and is often with intravenous cotrimoxazole in high doses (e.g. trimethoprim 20 mg/kg/day). Myelosuppression leads to discontinuation of therapy. Pentamidine, given intravenously, is an alternative form of treatment although toxic side effects (hypoglycaemia, hypokalaemia, hypotension and abnormal liver function tests) limit its usefulness. Inhaled pentamidine has been used in the acute phase in adults with good results.

Secondary prophylaxis must be instituted if the child survives one attack of PCP. Guidelines for primary prophylaxis state that children with CD4 counts which are persistently <400 cells/mm^3 should also be given primary prophylaxis against PCP. Drugs which are of proven benefit include trimethoprim and inhaled pentamidine, although the exact dosages and frequency of administration have not yet been established.

Protozoal infections

The child with protracted diarrhoea should be evaluated for the presence of bacterial and viral enteritides, as well as for protozoal infections. An empirical course of metronidazole may eradicate *Giardia lamblia*. Infection with cryptosporidium is refractory to treatment, and drugs which can be tried include spiramycin, erythromycin or clindamycin. Diarrhoea caused by *Isospora belli* may respond to cotrimoxazole.

Infection of the central nervous system with *Toxoplasma gondii* is rare in children. In adults, treatment is with pyrimethamine and sulphadiazine. Other drugs include clindamycin and trimethexate. Treatment is usually for an indefinite period due to frequent relapses, although it may be possible to reduce the dosage and frequency of treatment during maintenance.

Respiratory symptoms

Pulmonary infiltrates on the chest X-ray carry a wide differential diagnosis which may vary from acute bacterial pneumonia to lymphoid interstitial pneumonitis. On the other hand, the chest X-ray could be normal in a child with symptoms. The clinical picture together with evidence of immune compromise might be helpful in guiding treatment, but many infants are diagnosed with *Pneumocystis carinii* pneumonia as the first presentation of HIV disease in the family. In areas where the prevalence of HIV is high, clinicians must be alert to this diagnosis and start appropriate therapy empirically and promptly.

The drug regime used in PCP has already been discussed, and is usually insufficient on its own. Oxygen therapy is required, either via a head box in young infants, or face mask in older children. With the onset of acute respiratory failure, mechanical ventilation has to be considered. The prognosis for children who require mechanical ventilation is poor, with a median survival of one month compared to ten months for those children who survive PCP without mechanical ventilation. The parents' wishes must always be taken into consideration when deciding on such aggressive intervention, as the long-term outlook is poor.

Lymphoid interstitial pneumonia (LIP) usually carries a much better prognosis, with an overall mortality of 14 per cent. There is, however, considerable morbidity with chronic respiratory symptoms, hypoxaemia and congestive cardiac failure. The natural history of this condition is as yet undefined, although spontaneous resolution of radiological findings can occur without specific therapy. Children with LIP can also present acutely with an infectious episode. Repeated acute respiratory infections warrant several courses of antibiotics. Chronic hypoxaemia leads to limited exercise tolerance and supplemental oxygen may be needed, either on an intermittent or continuous basis. With the help of the home care team, families can cope with home oxygen therapy.

The use of corticosteroids has been advocated, although there is concern about steroid therapy in a child who may already be immune compromised. Anecdotal reports of good response to zidovudine therapy also exist, and placebo-controlled trials are awaited.

Central nervous system involvement

Neurological symptoms in children are more often attributable to HIV infection rather than other infections, malignancy, or cerebrovascular accidents. It is, however, wise to perform a lumbar puncture to exclude bacterial or cryptococcal meningitis, as well as Computerised Axial Tomography (CAT) or Magnetic Resonance Imaging (MRI) to rule out toxoplasmosis, brain abscesses, cerebral haemorrhages or lymphoma.

Sequential assessments and measurements of head size will reveal delays or regression in development. Neurological symptoms can progress at various speeds, remaining static in some children. The ultimate outlook is a child with multiple handicaps caused by impaired brain growth, loss or failure to achieve cognitive skills and motor milestones. (See also Chapter 10.)

The multidisciplinary model, used in the care of children with cerebral palsy, can be applied to the management of children with HIV encephalopathy. Apart from clinicians, assessment and intervention are required from the physiotherapist, clinical psychologist, occupational therapist, speech therapist and staff from special educational services. The family will require assistance from the Social Work Department for adaptations or modifications to the home and school in order to accommodate the handicapped child.

Encouraging results have been reported[11] on the use of zidovudine in children with neurological signs and symptoms. Cognitive function was improved even in those children without overt neurological involvement. The long term effects of therapy are not yet known.

Other therapies

Immune thrombocytopenia may be asymptomatic, requiring no active intervention. Usually, when the platelet count falls $<20 \times 10^9/L$, spontaneous bruising and bleeding occurs. Treatment with steroids, splenectomy and high dose intravenous immunoglobulin have been tried with limited success. Zidovudine may have a place in increasing platelet counts.

During end-stage disease, there may be coagulation problems and marrow failure. Blood product support may be necessary, and the use of CMV negative blood has been recommended together with irradiated blood to prevent graft-versus-host disease.

Anti-retroviral therapy

Each stage of viral replication serves as a potential target for therapy. Most agents have focussed on the enzyme reverse transcriptase, with zidovudine (3'-azido-2',3' dideoxythymidine) the best known and the only drug licensed for use at present. Several phase 1 studies have been completed in children, with proven efficacy[12]. Regimes have varied from continuous intravenous administration (0.9–1.4 mg/kg/hr), through intermittent intravenous therapy (80–160 mg/m^2, 6 hourly) to oral dosage (120–240 mg/m^2, 6 hourly). Zidovudine appears to have manageable toxic effects, including anaemia, neutropenia, nausea, abdominal discomfort, disturbed sleep and headaches which resolve either spontaneously or with dose reduction.

While the use of zidovudine in ill children is not disputed, guidelines for initiating therapy in those with mild or asymptomatic disease do not exist. In adults, zidovudine has been administered to patients with asymptomatic HIV infection, but who have <500 CD4 cells/mm^{3,13}. Compared to patients on placebo, those on active treatment showed a significant reduction in the rate of progression of disease. Although a low dose of zidovudine was found to be efficacious, the overall benefit of early intervention must be weighed against potential toxicity, the development of resistant strains of HIV, the costs of therapy and the uncertainty that long term benefits are conferred to children.

Other anti-retroviral agents with reported efficacy are the purine analogues 2',3' dideoxyinosine (ddI) and 2',3' dideoxycytidine (ddC). Phase 1 trials have been completed in adults using ddI, which show anti-retroviral activity with clinical improvement and diminished levels of serum HIV antigen levels. Side effects include pancreatitis and peripheral neuropathy.

Trials are also ongoing using soluble CD4 antigen in an attempt to stop viral entry into cells. At present, therapy is administered either intramuscularly or by subcutaneous infusion. Much work requires to be performed on the efficacy and toxicity of the newer anti-retroviral drugs in multi-centre, controlled clinical trials before they can be released for routine use. The ultimate aim would be to develop a regime which promises maximal efficacy with minimal toxic effects, by using a combination of drugs along the lines of anti-cancer therapy. [See manufacturers' literature for the most recent information regarding dosages, contraindications and side effects. Ed.]

Terminal care

The natural history of HIV disease in children remains undefined, so that families of infected children live with anxiety and uncertainty about their child's future. With time, and with each hospital admission, parents come to realise that the illness may be terminal.

Acute illness in an index case

A diagnosis of *Pneumocystis carinii* pneumonia in an infant usually leads to investigations which reveal that the infant is also HIV-infected, together with the mother and other members of the family. The family have then to come to terms with the shock of a seriously ill child, as well as the traumas of being an HIV-infected family. With little background information on the child's immune status, and less insight into the ultimate outlook for the child, the paediatrician must discuss various options with the family. Antimicrobial and supportive therapy must be instituted, and most parents under these circumstances will want all possible active treatment for the child, including assisted ventilation.

Chronic illness

The extended family may be alienated because of drug use, or not informed of the diagnosis of HIV. Either way, grandparents may be excluded from the sharing of experiences during the child's terminal illness. Tragically, some children have watched their own parents, siblings or close relatives die with AIDS as they go through their own illness. Depending on the age of the child, the responsible adults have to decide whether and what he or she has to be told. Support must be obtained from professionals experienced in dealing with dying children, to help children talk through their fears and anxieties.

Finally, when no further medical intervention is possible, parents have to decide if they wish to nurse the child in hospital, in a hospice, or at home. Parents have to be part of any decision made during the final stages of their child's illness, and a prime concern is that the child is free from pain. Again, paediatricians who have experience in the palliative care of oncology patients should be consulted on the care regime. The paediatrician or other clinician who has been responsible for the long term care of the child and family is best placed to manage the terminal illness, with the help and advice from other colleagues. Every effort should be made to ensure that the parents are present at the time of death. The doctor certifying the death must be sensitive in ensuring that the final stigma of AIDS does not appear on the death certificate. Practical assistance regarding funeral arrangements must be given, as the parents may not have had previous experience of the death of a child. Following the child's death, regular telephone contact or visits to the home let the families know that they have not been forgotten. (See also Chapters 7, 11 and 12.)

Immunisations

Theoretical arguments exist as to why live vaccines should not be given to individuals infected with HIV. These have not withstood results of retrospective or prospective reviews, and indeed, recommendations from the World Health Organisation are that live vaccines should be given to all HIV-infected individuals, with the exception of BCG in the patients with symptomatic disease.

In the United Kingdom, the Joint Committee on Vaccination and Immunisation recommend that inactivated vaccines (diphtheria, tetanus, pertussis) should be administered to all children. Live vaccines (polio, measles, mumps, rubella) are also considered safe for asymptomatic HIV-infected children. Indeed, there are good grounds to complete the course of primary immunisation as early as feasible, prior to the onset of immune deficiency.

Caution may have to be exercised in the use of oral polio vaccine. Although this is safe for infected children, other infected family members might be previously unvaccinated and at risk of complications of live polio vaccination. The excretion of the vaccine virus in the faeces of an immune compromised child may last for several months, so that parents should be advised on thorough handwashing after they change the infant's nappies. Because of these problems, some clinicians may choose to use inactivated polio vaccine. Table 3.5 outlines recommendations on the use of vaccines in HIV-infected

Table 3.5   Recommendations on vaccination of HIV-infected children

Vaccine	WHO Asyx/Syx		JCVI (UK) Asyx/Syx		ACIP (USA) Asyx/Syx	
BCG	+	–	–	–	–	–
DTP	+	+	+	+	+	+
OPV	+	+	*	*	*	*
IPV	+	+	+	+	+	+
Measles	+	+	Not available		+	+
MMR	+	+	+	+	+	–
HBV	+	+	+	+	+	+
Pneumococcal	–	+	–	–	–	+
Influenza	–	+	–	–	–	+

WHO, World Health Organisation. JCVI, Joint Committee on Vaccination and Immunisation. ACIP, Advisory Committee on Immunisation Practices. *, Discretion of clinician, depending on other infected family members. Asyx = Asymptomatic. Syx = Symptomatic.

children. Most authorities advise that the clinical and immunological status of the child should be considered.

Despite immunisation, suboptimal responses to the vaccine may be obtained. Antibody levels to the vaccine will have to be monitored, and in the absence of a response, passive immunisation must be given following known contact with measles or chickenpox. The families of symptomatic children should be encouraged to report promptly any known contact with childhood infectious diseases so the paediatrician can decide on the appropriate therapy, which is usually effective only if given early. For measles contact, hyperimmune human globulin may be available and needs to be administered as soon as possible.

Contact with chickenpox or shingles merits administration of human varicella zoster immunoglobulin (VZIG) within 10 days of exposure, followed by the careful monitoring for clinical disease. Even with prompt administration of VZIG within 72 hours of contact, infection is not prevented but the disease is attenuated. Appearance of chickenpox lesions in the immune suppressed child warrants acyclovir therapy.

Prognosis

Children with AIDS who were reported to the Centers for Disease Control in the United States survived a median of nine months following diagnosis and 75 per cent had died within two years[14]. Follow-up has not been long enough to obtain a true estimate of mortality, and advances in the management of HIV-infected children will improve survival rates. It is known that the age of the child and type of disease presentation influences survival, with the poorest prognosis seen in those children aged under one year who present with an opportunistic infection. In developing countries, other infectious complications and malnutrition contribute to the high mortality seen amongst HIV-infected children.

Scott and her co-workers in Miami[15] described seven common patterns of clinical disease – PCP, *Candida* oesophagitis, LIP, recurrent bacterial infection, cardiomyopathy, encephalopathy and renal disease – in a cohort of HIV-infected children, 91 per cent of whom were black, and who had all been infected vertically. Differences were seen in the age of diagnosis as well as in survival time following diagnosis. PCP and encephalopathy developed in very young children (median age five and nine months respectively) while nephropathy was diagnosed much later (median age 39 months). Median survival was also influenced by disease pattern and was one month for PCP and 72 months for LIP.

Many longitudinal studies are highlighting the fact that the age distribution for HIV disease is bimodal, even within the paediatric population (see Chapter 1). Survival from the onset of clinical disease depends on many factors which have not been elucidated. Also, the role of co-factors are unknown either in the development of clinical disease or in the rate of disease progression. Identification of infected children and regular monitoring are of utmost importance, as early diagnosis allows for prompt intervention before the onset of progressive disease.

References

1. Marion, R. W., Wiznia, A. A., Hutcheon, G., Rubinstein, A. (1986). Human T-cell lymphotropic virus type III embryopathy. *American Journal of Diseases of Children*, **140**, 638–40.
2. Epstein, L. G., Sharer, L. R., Oleske, J. M. *et al.* (1986). Neurologic manifestations of human immunodeficiency virus infection in children. *Pediatrics*, **78**, 678–87.
3. Belman, A. L., Diamond, G. W., Dickson, D. *et al.* (1988). Pediatric acquired immunodeficiency syndrome: neurological syndromes. *Journal of Diseases in Children*, **142**, 29–35.
4. European Collaborative Study (1990). Neurologic signs in young children with HIV infection. *Pediatric Infectious Diseases Journal*, **9**, 402–6.
5. Rubinstein, A., Morecki, R., Silverman, B. *et al.* (1986). Pulmonary disease in children with AIDS and AIDS related complex. *Journal of Pediatrics*, **108**, 498–503.
6. Joshi, V. V., Kauffman, S., Oleske, J. M. *et al.* (1987). Polyclonal polymorphic B cell lymphoproliferative disorder with prominant pulmonary involvement in children with AIDS. *Cancer*, **59**, 1455–62.
7. Borkowsky, W., Steele, C. J., Grubman, S. *et al.* (1987). Antibody responses to bacterial toxoids in children with HIV. *Journal of Pediatrics*, **110**, 563–6.
8. Bernstein, L. J., Ochs, H. D., Wedgwood, R. J., Rubinstein, A. (1985). Defective humoral immunity in pediatric AIDS. *Journal of Pediatrics*, **107**, 352–7.
9. Mok, J., Hague, R. A., Taylor, R. F. *et al.* (1989). The management of infants born to HIV seropositive women. *Journal of Infection*, **18**, 119–24.
10. Hague, R. A., Burns, S., Mok, J., Yap, P. L. (1990). Diagnosis of *Pneumocystis carinii* pneumonia from non-invasive sampling of respiratory secretions. *Archives of Disease in Childhood*, **65**, 1364–5.
11. Pizzo, P. A., Eddy, J., Falloon, J. *et al.* (1988). Effect of continuous intravenous infusion of Zidovudine (AZT) in children with symptomatic HIV infection. *New England Journal of Medicine*, **319**, 889–96.
12. McKinney, R. E., Pizzo, P. A., Scott, G. B. *et al.* (1990). Safety and tolerance of intermittent intravenous and oral Zidovudine therapy in HIV-infected pediatric patients. *American Journal of Diseases of Children*, **140**, 638–40.
13. Volberding, P. A., Lagakos, S. W., Koch, M. A. *et al.* (1990). Zidovudine in asymptomatic HIV infection. A controlled trial in persons with fewer than 500 CD4-positive cells/mm^3. *New England Journal of Medicine*, **322**, 941–9.
14. Rogers, M. F., Thomas, P. A., Starcher, E. A. *et al.* (1987). AIDS in children: report of the Centers for Disease Control national surveillance, 1982–1985. *Pediatrics*, **79**, 1008–14.

15. Scott, G. B., Hutto, C., Makuch, R. W. *et al.* (1989). Survival in children with perinatally acquired HIV type 1 infection. *New England Journal of Medicine*, **321**, 1791–6.

4 Part 1 The care and management of children with haemophilia and HIV infection

Mark Winter

History of haemophilia

The genetic mutation that is the cause of haemophilia is probably very old as it can be found in at least three orders of placental mammals; as well as man, haemophilia is also known to occur in both the horse and the dog[1]. Several references to children with a history of easy bruising are to be found in the Babylonian Talmud of the second century AD.

Many people are aware of haemophilia through its association with Queen Victoria and her family. The Queen's eighth child, the Duke of Albany, was a severe haemophiliac and two of her daughters proved to be haemophilia carriers, transmitting the haemophilia gene into several European royal families. The destabilising effect that the severe haemophilia suffered by Prince Alexis (Queen Victoria's great-grandson) had on the Russian Royal Family, together with the relationship of the child to Rasputin, has been well documented[1].

The rather curious term 'haemophilia', literally 'the love of blood', was first used by Hopff in 1828. During the first half of the twentieth century, the idea evolved that haemophilia resulted from the lack of a clotting factor, which was referred to as 'antihaemophilic globulin'. Subsequently, this protein became known as Factor VIII.

In 1947, Pavlovsky showed that it was possible to mutually correct the abnormal clotting times of some haemophiliac blood samples by mixing them together[2]. This observation suggested that there might be more than one type of haemophilia and in 1956 a Canadian patient from Oxford was described as having a form of haemophilia that was not due to Factor VIII deficiency. This disorder was originally known as Christmas disease (the paper appeared in the Christmas edition of the *British Medical Journal* and also happened to be the patient's surname), but it is now known universally as Factor IX deficiency.

The process of blood coagulation is a very complex one in which a series of clotting factors are activated, eventually leading to the production of fibrin. The clinical disorder of haemophilia can result from the lack of any one of these clotting factors, although in practice most patients prove to have either a deficiency of Factor VIII or Factor IX. Thus, at the end of 1989, there were more than 5,000 patients with Factor VIII deficiency and 1,000 patients with Factor IX deficiency known to be registered at British Haemophilia Centres.

Inheritance

Deficiencies of both Factor VIII and IX are inherited according to an X-linked recessive pattern (see Fig. 4.1). In effect, this will mean that all the daughters of a haemophiliac will be carriers whereas all of the sons (who must inherit their father's Y chromosome rather than the abnormal X chromosome) will be normal. Furthermore, we can say that there is a one in two chance that the son of a haemophilia carrier will be affected and similarly a one in two chance that the daughter of a haemophilia carrier will carry the haemophilia gene. In some families, where there is no history of haemophilia, it is likely that the abnormal gene has arisen as a result of a new mutation. With the advent of recombinant DNA technology, it has been possible to clone the Factor VIII gene and to use selective probes to investigate the specific genetic abnormalities occurring in haemophiliac families. A few such patients have now been shown to have partial deletions or specific mutations of the Factor VIII gene, each abnormality being unique to each family[3].

Similarly, DNA technology has resulted in the development of several intra-genic probes which not only permit the detection of the haemophilia carrier state[4] but also offer the possibility of diagnosing haemophilia *in utero*[5]; antenatal diagnosis now being possible at the gestation age of eight weeks onwards through chorion villus sampling.

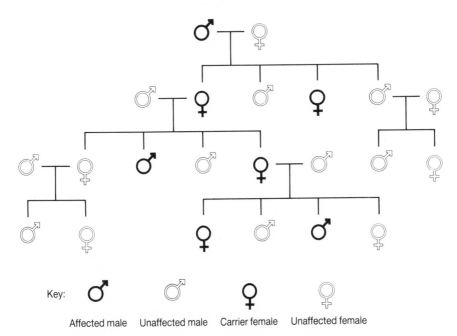

Fig. 4.1 Mode of inheritance of haemophilia. Reproduced with kind permission of the Haemophilia Society, London.

Clinical features of haemophilia

It is not widely understood that the clinical features of bleeding in haemophilia are usually restricted to deep-seated tissues such as joints and muscles. In particular, it is important to realise that haemophiliacs do not bleed excessively following trivial lacerations to the skin; nor is there an increased tendency towards bleeding from mucous membranes. These observations will be particularly relevant when we come to stress how unlikely it is that an HIV-positive haemophiliac will be an infectious risk in a school setting. These clinical findings can be explained on the basis that haemostasis in small vessels, such as those which predominate in skin and mucous membranes, is mediated predominantly by platelets. That traditional clinical test of haemostasis 'the bleeding time' (which sounds as if it ought to be prolonged in haemophilia) is in practice normal, as it depends mainly on platelet number and function as well as on the presence of a protein known as Von Willebrand factor; it is not dependent on the presence of clotting factors. In contrast, the coagulation pathways leading to the formation of fibrin appear to be more involved in haemostasis as it occurs in larger vessels, such as those which are to be found in joints and muscles.

In summary, patients with platelet pathology (for example, children with leukaemia) will tend to suffer from skin and mucous membrane bleeding, whereas patients with coagulation factor deficiencies (such as haemophiliacs) will be more likely to bleed into major organs such as joints and muscles. However, it should also be noted that haemophiliac bleeding may occur into any internal organ, with particularly grave consequences if, for instance, the brain is involved.

A further important clinical difference between 'platelet' bleeding and 'clotting factor' bleeding is that the patient with either absent or defective platelets will bleed almost immediately following trauma, as it is the function of platelets to induce the process known as primary haemostasis which is mediated by platelet adhesion and aggregation. The role of the coagulation pathway is to synthesise fibrin, which in turn supports the primary platelet plug. As a result, a haemophiliac experiencing trauma will not bleed immediately as platelet function is not impaired and primary haemostasis can be achieved. However, the fibrin plug cannot be formed and the platelet plug, being unsupported, eventually breaks down with resultant bleeding. A characteristic history of an episode of bleeding in a haemophiliac child would consist of an apparently trivial traumatic event followed several hours later by the clinical signs of a bleed.

The most common and distressing symptom of severe haemophilia is recurrent bleeding into joints, particularly those of the lower limbs. If untreated, these episodes can lead quite readily to a vicious circle of bleeding causing joint damage, which in turn makes further bleeding more likely. As well as being a severe irritant, the presence of blood in the joint causes inevitable and irreversible damage to the articular surfaces and progressive destruction of articular cartilage. A particular feature of the latter process is the formation of hypertrophic fronds of cartilage which are especially fragile and prone to bleed. All this is compounded by the inevitable immobility that accompanies a serious joint bleed; the muscles surrounding the affected joint develop signs of disuse atrophy and result in a lack of stabilisation of an already pathologically abnormal joint. All these factors will tend to promote further episodes of bleeding.

Clinically, there are several different types of haemophilia depending on the relative lack of Factor VIII (or IX). Mildly affected patients will tend to bleed only after significant trauma, such as a surgical procedure or road traffic accident. Joint bleeds are very rare. Moderately affected patients will often bleed into joints and muscles after fairly trivial episodes of trauma, whereas most bleeds occurring in severely affected patients are likely to arise spontaneously.

Treatment of haemophilia

Prior to 1965 there was no effective means of concentrating Factor VIII from whole blood and the only treatment likely to be offered consisted of infusions of plasma combined with bed rest. In that year, Pool and Shannon reported from California the significant discovery that slow thawing at low temperature of fresh frozen plasma resulted in the formation of so-called cryoprecipitate ('formed in the cold') which was found to be rich in Factor VIII[6]. Here at last was a means of obtaining Factor VIII in amounts that were of genuine benefit to haemophiliacs. The discovery of cryopreciptate is now regarded as a landmark in the treatment of haemophilia, but it was by no means an ideal form of therapy:

- It was cumbersome and time consuming to prepare.
- It had to be stored at −20°C and was thus not suitable for home therapy.
- The exact amount of Factor VIII in each bag was not known.
- The final volume for injection was often large enough to be a problem if the patient was a child or in heart failure.

What was needed was a concentrate of Factor VIII that could be kept in a domestic refrigerator, that dissolved in a small volume and in which the number of units of Factor VIII was known. These concentrates, now so familiar to haemophiliac patients and their families, eventually became available in the early 1970s.

The advent of Factor VIII and IX concentrates was followed rapidly by the development of home therapy programmes and the whole pattern of haemophilia care changed dramatically. Patients relished their new found independence and their lives no longer revolved around pathology laboratories and out-patient departments[7]. The parents of children as young as four or five could be taught how to inject Factor VIII and these children could then start to attend mainstream schools. As the effect of a Factor VIII infusion only lasts for a few hours, most patients only treated themselves when they bled (demand therapy), although if recurrent bleeding into one joint became a problem the patients would be asked to inject three times weekly (prophylactic therapy). Not only the quality of life, but life expectancy itself, changed dramatically[8]. The concept of comprehensive haemophilia care emerged – the patient would be seen at regular intervals for review, including orthopaedic assessments, dental care, social welfare and counselling together with clinical and laboratory assessment of his haemophilia.

Complications of haemophilia therapy

Despite the obvious significant advantages associated with the introduction of Factor concentrates, it was nevertheless apparent that there were important problems that could seriously affect patients with haemophilia. Firstly, a number of patients (usually between 5–15 per cent in most studies) could be shown to develop an inhibitor against Factor VIII. This complication frequently led to a lack of response to even high doses of infused concentrates and other more complex therapies, such as activated Factor IX concentrates or porcine Factor VIII[9], were often needed to control episodes of bleeding.

Secondly, and of great consequence when we come to discuss HIV infection in haemophilia, it soon became apparent that the concentrates could contain and could transmit various forms of hepatitis[10]. About 10 per cent of regularly treated haemophiliacs were found to be carriers of hepatitis B and about 50 per cent were assumed to have been exposed to hepatitis B as their blood contained antibody against hepatitis B surface antigen. In addition, a significant number of patients displaying abnormalities of liver function had no markers of infection with either hepatitis A or B and were assumed to have 'non-A, non-B hepatitis'. Recently, this virus (now termed hepatitis C) has been putatively identified and an antibody test developed[11]. Although the onset of this form of hepatitis is usually sub-clinical, there is recent evidence to suggest that with time many patients with haemophilia are likely to develop serious chronic liver disease[12].

The advent of the HIV epidemic in haemophilia

The first cases of AIDS occurring in haemophiliacs were reported in 1982[13] more than a year after the original descriptions of the disorder. Early theories on the aetiology of the immune suppression that was clearly the hallmark of AIDS included speculation that there were factors in the homosexual life-style, perhaps the use of amyl nitrites for instance, that were responsible for the development of the syndrome. However, the emerging number of haemophiliacs and transfusion recipients with AIDS provided definite evidence for the presence of a transmissible agent.

Following the original isolation of the virus that became known as HIV[14] serological tests rapidly became available[15]. Only at this time did the profound impact that HIV was to have on the lives of haemophiliacs become apparent. It appeared that the vast majority of regularly treated haemophiliacs, as high as 90 per cent in some centres, would prove to be HIV-antibody positive. For instance, a 1987 survey by the UK Haemophilia Directors Organisation[16] showed that 782 out of 1,333 severely affected patients (59%) tested positive. How could this tragic situation have occurred?

Each batch of Factor VIII concentrate is prepared from the plasma of a large number of donors, usually at least 5,000 and often as many as 20,000. Herein lies the reason for the high incidence of HIV infection in haemophiliacs for, in theory, the presence of the virus in the plasma of just one donor could lead to most or all recipients of that batch becoming infected. As it was inevitable that patients were treated with many different batches every year the chances of infection were exceedingly high. The contrast between receiving Factor VIII concentrates and a blood transfusion is very significant in this respect. For instance, a patient given four units of blood to cover a gastrectomy would be exposed to any viruses present in the blood of only four donors, whereas each time a haemophiliac receives treatment (usually 30–50 times each year) he is potentially exposed to the viruses of many thousands of donors. In the former situation the chance of viral infection is very low; in the latter, it is very high.

Traditionally, haemophiliacs have been treated in the UK with a combination of NHS Factor VIII (prepared from volunteer donor plasma) and commercial Factor VIII concentrates. Unlike some other countries, the political decision to become self-sufficient in blood and blood products was never taken, even though there was strong evidence to suppose that because commercial concentrates were prepared from the plasma of paid donors they were inherently more likely to transmit infectious viruses. The incidence of HIV infection in haemophiliacs proved to be much lower in those countries that had become self-sufficient, although it should be noted that no form of Factor VIII proved to be safe. Some haemophiliacs who received exclusively NHS Factor VIII concentrate still sero-converted and produced antibodies to HIV.

Some Haemophilia Centres had been in the habit of freezing and storing samples of their patients' blood on a long term basis. These frozen samples provided valuable information concerning the onset of HIV infection in haemophiliacs, as it could be shown that in retrospect most patients had sero-converted between 1981 and 1983.

Making Factor VIII safer

Because of the already apparent problem with hepatitis, several commercial companies introduced trials of heat treated Factor VIII in the early 1980s. Although only of limited success in the removal of hepatitis viruses, it appeared that heat treatment was very effective at breaking down HIV. From July 1984 onwards, all haemophiliacs were changed over to exclusively heat treated products. Currently, there are several types of heat treated concentrate available depending on whether the heat is applied when the concentrate is in the form of a 'dry' powder (as in NHS Factor VIII) or in the form of a 'wet' slurry (most commercial companies). Although it looks as if heat treatment of 'wet' Factor VIII is more effective in removing the various hepatitis viruses, fortunately all forms of heat treated concentrates currently available seem to be highly effective in preventing HIV transmission. Many haemophiliac children, born since 1984, have been treated with these newer concentrates and have remained HIV-negative.

Other measures were also taken to promote increased safety of concentrates. The selection of donors by commercial companies became more rigorously controlled and all donors were screened for HIV. As well as Factor VIII, *all* donated blood in the UK has been screened for HIV-1 since October 1985.

The future of blood products

There is current controversy as to whether further tests should be used in the screening of all blood donors. Under active consideration at this time, and already implemented by companies, are assays for the following:

- HTLV I: A retrovirus, in some ways similar to HIV, which causes a form of T cell leukaemia. The virus is particularly common amongst peoples of West Indian and Oriental extraction.
- Hepatitis C: This test is likely to be introduced once methodological problems have been resolved.
- Anti-hepatitis B core: This antibody has been called a 'surrogate' marker as it seems to be associated with patients who are likely to have hepatitis C.
- ALT (Alanine transaminase): This will detect any donors with hepatic inflammation, such as hepatitis.

- HIV-2: Already found in other parts of the world, recently introduced in France. Some HIV-2 positive patients have been identified in the UK. (See also Chapter 2.)

As well as understandable concerns about the safety of Factor VIII there is also increasing interest in making the concentrates more 'pure' as they are known to contain irrelevant proteins which may cause immunosuppression. In particular, two recent developments include:

- solvent detergent Factor VIII[17]: a combination of TNBP (tri-n-butyl phosphate) and polysorbates has been shown to inactivate viruses without having any effect on protein structure or function.
- monoclonal Factor VIII[18]: Factor VIII is concentrated by binding to a column-associated antibody to part of the Factor VIII molecule. This process results in a highly purified form of Factor VIII concentrate.

Whilst we continue to rely on Factor VIII that has been derived from blood donors, there remains a risk that haemophiliacs will acquire significant viral infections from these concentrates. The way forward lies with genetic engineering, for it has now proved possible to clone the gene that synthesises Factor VIII[19]. This 'recombinant' Factor VIII is now in clinical trial and appears to be both safe and effective in controlling episodes of bleeding[20]. For those countries with poorly developed blood donation programmes, recombinant Factor VIII will offer the only realistic hope of effective therapy for thousands of haemophiliacs in the developing world.

The main problem is likely to be financial – how are we to afford this treatment for our patients? Should we strive to use the more expensive recombinant Factor VIII, or bow to economic pressures and use cheaper products such as heat treated Factor VIII? The answer is surely provided by the example of what happened when Factor VIII concentrates were not as safe as they should have been. How do we know that there is not another virus like HIV already present in our concentrates that is waiting to be discovered? For the past seven years, everyone concerned with haemophilia – patients, families and carers – has lived through a series of crises as the extent of the HIV problem has become apparent. The least that can be done now is to make sure that our patients get the best, safest and purest Factor VIII that there is. At least that will minimise the chances that this sort of problem will ever have to be faced again.

Haemophiliac children with HIV

A survey by the UK Haemophilia Directors Organisation[16] showed that there were 293 haemophiliac children and teenagers reported as being HIV

Table 4.1 Number of haemophiliac children and teenagers reported as HIV antibody positive

Age	Patients tested	Patients positive
5	122	13
5–9	226	52
10–14	249	97
15–19	308	131

antibody positive in 1986. (It should be noted that only 79 per cent of centres responded.) (See Table 4.1.)

Treatment and follow-up for children with HIV and haemophilia

The medical follow-up of HIV-positive children has been extensively discussed in Chapter 3. The effective management of HIV-positive haemophiliacs involves appreciation of the profound and highly significant differences between these patients and other children with HIV – in the clinical disorders from which they may suffer, the interpretation of prognostic markers, the investigation of possible AIDS-related pathologies and the medical treatment of the condition. These critical differences, sadly sometimes either ignored or misunderstood by many centres, will more often than not lead to disastrous consequences if the haemophiliac child is managed in a unit that is inexperienced in haemophilia care. Furthermore, haemophiliac HIV is different because the child has a pre-existing disorder and it is inevitable that HIV infection will have a demonstrable effect on the state of the patient's haemophilia. It is also possible in theory that treatment of the child's haemophilia may promote progression of HIV disease.

Clinical differences

There is clear evidence for a different pattern of HIV pathology in haemophiliacs:

- Kaposi's sarcoma occurs extremely rarely, if at all, in patients who were infected with HIV following the use of blood products.
- There is a growing impression that haemophiliacs may be more likely to suffer from non-Hodgkins lymphoma, particularly from aggressive and clinically atypical forms involving the bone marrow and central nervous system.
- There is an increased incidence of severe thrombocytopenia in HIV-positive haemophiliacs. The aetiology of the low platelet count that can be associated with HIV is thought to be primarily auto-immune in origin. As more regularly treated haemophiliacs will have chronic liver disease (following infection with hepatitis viruses) the increased tendency towards thrombocytopenia could be explicable on the basis that their platelet counts are also being suppressed by hypersplenism secondary to chronic liver pathology.

Differences in prognostic markers

- CD4 (T4) levels: although regular assessment of CD4 levels may remain of benefit and yield important prognostic information, it should be noted that HIV-negative haemophiliacs may also have low levels[21]. The immunosuppression observed in regularly treated haemophiliacs, which may prove to have important clinical consequences, is likely to be related to chronic exposure to the many different antigens present in Factor VIII concentrates.
- β2 microglobulin: this protein is a marker of immune activation and it is said that increased levels may correlate with progression to AIDS.

However, haemophiliacs may already have elevated levels from the antigenic stimulation that accompanies regular concentrate therapy.
• LDH: raised levels of lactate dehydrogenase have been suggested to be a marker of pneumocystis infection but levels are likely to be already elevated in the majority of regularly treated haemophiliacs.

Differences in diagnostic techniques

Invasive techniques are accepted as having an established place in the diagnosis of pathologies related to HIV. For example, a patient might require a bronchoscopy for the diagnosis of pneumocystis, or a lymph node biopsy for the detection of lymphoma. These routine investigations represent a far more difficult undertaking for the haemophiliac with his profound bleeding tendency. Not only will the patient require high doses of Factor VIII on a daily basis, but assays of circulating Factor VIII will be needed (to ensure adequate haemostasis) as well as pre-operative investigations to exclude an inhibitor to Factor VIII. All this is likely to result in the haemophiliac being in hospital for two to three times as long as other patients.

Differences in management and treatment

Similarly, any operation required, for example, a splenectomy for idiopathic thrombocytopenic purpura, which would be regarded as routine in normal circumstances, becomes a major undertaking with undoubted excess morbidity.

Any physician caring for these patients will also need to consider the background of the child's haemophilia. For instance, if the child already has a low platelet count (due to chronic liver disease) the introduction of anti-retroviral drugs such as AZT (zidovudine), which are known to cause potential bone marrow suppression, will have to be carefully monitored. Anti-platelet agents, such as aspirin and ibuprofen, are strictly contra-indicated in haemophilia as they will cause an increased risk of haemorrhage; this must be borne in mind when prescribing analgesics, anti-inflammatory and anti-pyretic agents. Finally, under normal circumstances it is advisable for haemophiliacs not to receive intramuscular injections because of the risk of haematoma formation.

The impact of HIV on haemophilia

It must be expected that there will be a dynamic relationship between the two lifelong illnesses the child now suffers – haemophilia and HIV infection. Each disorder may have a profound effect on the nature of the pathology in the other disorder. For example, over the past few years there has been a striking increase in the incidence of septic arthritis in haemophilia[22]. This is highly likely to be related to HIV-associated immunosuppression in this group of patients. There is also some evidence that Factor VIII requirements are increasing in HIV-positive haemophiliacs. In part, this could be explained by any depression of the platelet count (by either HIV itself or various therapies) leading to increased bleeding. Factor VIII will also be required in increased amounts as the child becomes ill and investigations and treatments are planned.

The impact of haemophilia on HIV

Does haemophilia or its treatment have any effect on the rate of progression of HIV? The answer is not known at present, but in theory regular Factor VIII therapy could cause immunosuppression because of the large amounts of contaminant proteins to which the haemophiliac is exposed. There is an urgent need to find out whether this depression of immune function is clinically relevant; if so, there will be a clear case for giving the highly purified monoclonal concentrates to all those infected with HIV.

Progression of HIV infection in haemophiliac children

Originally it was hoped that the proportion of haemophiliacs who would develop AIDS would be less than other patients as the virus had been freeze dried during the preparation of the Factor VIII and therefore possibly attenuated. Unfortunately, it is now accepted that there is no difference in the risk of developing AIDS in haemophiliacs.

Recent studies[23] indicate that there is a strong association between increasing age and the development of AIDS amongst haemophiliacs (see Table 4.2).

Table 4.2   Age and the development of AIDS amongst haemophiliacs

Age group	Cumulative incidence of AIDS five years after seroconversion (percentage)
<25	4
25–44	6
>44	19

Although the risk of AIDS may currently be relatively low for haemophiliac children, medical opinion suggests that with time most HIV-infected persons will eventually become unwell. For this reason, there is increasing interest in 'early intervention', including the use of anti-retroviral agents and prophylactic pentamidine (for the prevention of *Pneumocystis carinii* pneumonia) in asymptomatic patients.

Heterosexual transmission of HIV

One of the most difficult of the many problems that HIV-positive teenagers will have to learn to accept is that they may be able to pass on their HIV through sexual activity. At this time, most studies[24] indicate that around 10 per cent of sexual partners of HIV-positive haemophiliacs are likely to be infected. Although this is rather a lower figure than reported for sexual partners of non-haemophiliacs, it must be stated that the number of partners of haemophiliacs who have been infected is steadily increasing and the risk of transmission remains a very real one. According to some reports, the likelihood of transmission may be increased when the haemophiliac is HIV-antigen positive or when the CD4 count is severely reduced.

Talking to children about HIV

There is little doubt that some Haemophilia Centres have been reluctant to grasp the issue of talking to their children about HIV. Although in many ways understandable, this approach is in the author's view misguided and experience suggests that indeed it may make a difficult situation even worse.

By the spring of 1985 it was clear that the majority of the 27 haemophiliacs who had tested positive for HIV in our Centre were teenagers or children, the average age of the whole group being 19. Four of the patients were under eleven years of age and the youngest was six. The decision was taken that all of these young people would be told about their HIV at the appropriate time, provided that the parents were in agreement. Why was this done?

Reasons for telling children about HIV

Firstly, the child may already know or suspect that he has HIV. Children are sensitive to change and are very aware of their environment. They will doubtless have noticed that they are asked to visit the hospital more often and that when they arrive the doctors and nurses may look concerned. Sadly, it is also known that in some Centres when haemophiliacs are admitted to the hospital they are nursed in side wards by nursing staff using full barrier precautions. Although some parents have gone to great lengths to prevent their children from finding out about HIV, it seems inevitable that the child will eventually suspect that there is something desperately wrong. Unless checked, this can lead to a child's imagination running riot, especially if the child is made to wait outside in the corridor whilst the doctor talks to his parents.

Although telling a child that he has HIV might appear a dreadful ordeal, this need not necessarily be the case. The child is often 'ready to know' and indeed one of our young haemophiliacs had already asked his mother if he had been infected. Not only do children have a remarkable ability to come to terms with grief, it is also doubtless true that as adults we presume that our own concerns about HIV will prove to be the same as that of these children. This is a dangerous assumption; for the child the news might not invoke fears of becoming ill or dying but rather anxiety about missing school or not being able to play sport for instance. In any case, the child will have to be told eventually before he becomes sexually active. Although this 'delayed telling' may be favoured by some centres, it is likely that, for example, a fifteen-year-old boy who has been eventually told that he has had HIV for six years, will be not only upset but also angry that such information has been withheld from him for so long.

Should the school be told?

There is no formal obligation to tell a school about a child's HIV status and, indeed, many Haemophilia Centres have made a positive decision never to reveal this information. However, as the stigma of AIDS recedes and the prospect emerges of AIDS becoming a manageable chronic illness, might there now be a place for telling schools about HIV in the same way that one would about diabetes, epilepsy or cancer? There are certain advantages that might become apparent. The headteacher could take the child's HIV status into consideration when assessing progress, as would happen with other chronic and serious illnesses. Furthermore, there would be the comfort for the child of knowing that there was someone in the school who was aware of his problems and to whom he could turn whenever he was upset. We agreed with some of the parents of our HIV-positive children that two people in each school should be informed in this way, the headteacher and perhaps the form teacher. This practice has worked well in our Centre and the parents have been relieved that someone at the school knows all about the child's problems. There appears to have been no problems with confidentiality.

Helping the family

It is inevitable that the family, and all the dynamic relationships contained therein, will be profoundly affected by the child's HIV infection. Haemophilia itself presents a significant and stressful burden on every family. It is all too easy for the child's haemophilia to become the dominant factor in all their lives, with its sudden and painful episodes of unexpected bleeding often leading to cancellation of some planned family activity. Into this already pressurised situation has now been added all the difficulties that being HIV positive can bring. Anyone who has worked with people with AIDS will know of the intense spiritual and emotional problems that living with HIV presents. The bitterness and grief experienced by all patients can be even more poignant for children with haemophilia and their families.

Originally, before 1984–1985, there was expected to be a new generation of haemophiliacs; the first patients to receive proper treatment and to be free of chronic joint pain. Certainly it is true that, by and large, these children do have normal joints; but what has been so difficult to accept is that Factor VIII 'the very giver of life' has proved to take life away.

Health care staff should be aware that central to all the problems experienced by familes of haemophiliacs is the position of the mother. For many of these women there may be a profound sense of guilt for having passed on their haemophilia gene; they may well reason that their sons would not have been infected with HIV if they had not been carriers of haemophilia. For some of these mothers comes too the realisation that they may have actually injected the contaminated Factor VIII when the child received home therapy. There are many families in our Centre and elsewhere in which a mother has borne two (or more) sons, both of them haemophiliacs and both HIV-antibody positive.

Other members of the family also have reason to feel especially affected by the crisis. For the children who are not haemophiliacs there may be the feeling that they are being neglected, or they may feel 'survivors' guilt'; for the grandparents there can be the guilt that the haemophilia gene has been passed on through them.

There is no 'standard' way of responding to this myriad of problems. Many of our patients have learned to cope, albeit in different ways. For some, there is the comfort that religious belief can bring, whilst others find help and reassurance through our family support group. Some families spend much time talking to us at the Centre, whilst others keep their concerns to themselves until some event, such as the development of AIDS in a distant haemophiliac relative, or some form of media activity concerning HIV, provokes a torrent of repressed emotion.

The cornerstone of providing effective support for these people is not to consider the child, his haemophilia and his HIV in isolation, but rather to involve the family as a whole wherever possible. Each family should be regarded as a unique collection of individuals who happen to be related, all of them responding in a different way to the same crisis.

References

1. Ingram, G. I. C. (1976). A history of haemophilia. *Journal of Clinical Pathology*, **29**, 3–13.
2. Pavlovsky, A. (1947). Contribution to the pathogenesis of haemophilia. *Blood*, **2**, 185.
3. Antonarakis, S. E. (1988). The molecular genetics of haemophilia A and B in man. *Advances in Human Genetics*, **17**, 27–59.
4. Graham, J. B. (1990). Evolution of methods for carrier detection in haemophilia. *Progress in Clinical and Biological Research*, **324**, 29–38.
5. Koerper, M. A. (1990). Prenatal diagnosis of haemophilia in the United States. *Progress in Clinical and Biological Research*, **324**, 1–37.
6. Pool, J. D., Shannon, A. E. (1965). Production of high potency concentrates of antihaemophilic globulin in a closed bag system. *New England Journal of Medicine*, **273**, 1443–9.
7. Ingram, G. I. C., Dykes, S. R., Creese, A. L. (1979). Home treatment in haemophilia: clinical, social and economic advantages. *Clinical and Laboratory Haematology*, **I**, 13–27.
8. Smit, C., Rosendaal, F. R., Varekamp, I. (1989). Physical condition, longevity and social performance of Dutch haemophiliacs, 1972–85. *British Medical Journal*, **298**, 235–8.
9. Kernoff, P. B. A., Thomas, N. D., Lilley, P. A. *et al.* (1984). Clinical experience with polyelectrolyte – fractionated porcine Factor VIII concentrate in the treatment of haemophiliacs with antibodies to Factor VIII. *Blood*, **63**, 31–41.
10. Kasper, C. K., Kipnif, S. A. (1972). Hepatitis and clotting factor concentrates. *Journal of the American Medical Association*, **221**, 510.
11. Kuo, G., Choo, Q. L., Alter, H. J. (1989). An assay for circulating antibodies to a major aetiologic virus of human non-A, non-B hepatitis. *Science*, **244**, 362–4.
12. Hay, C. R. M., Preston, F. E., Triger, D. R., Underwood, J. C. E. (1985). Progressive liver disease in haemophilia: an understated problem? *Lancet*, **i**, 1495–8.
13. Centers for Disease Control (1982). Pneumocystis carinii pneumonia among persons with haemophilia A. *Morbidity and Mortality Weekly Report*, **31**, 365–7.
14. Barre-Sinoussi, F., Chermann, J.-C., Rey, F. (1983). Isolation of a T-lymphocytotrophic retrovirus from a patient at risk for acquired immunodeficiency syndrome. *Science*, **220**, 868–70.
15. Schupbach, J., Popovic, M., Gilden, R. V. *et al.* (1984). Serological analysis of a sub-group of human T-lymphocytotrophic retroviruses associated with AIDS. *Science*, **224**, 503–5.
16. AIDS group of the UK Haemophilia Centre Directors (1988). Prevalence of antibody to HIV in haemophiliacs in the United Kingdom. *Clinical and Laboratory Haematology*, **10**, 187–91.
17. Horowitz, B., Wiebe, M. E. (1985). Inactivation of viruses in labile blood derivatives. *Transfusion*, **25**, 516–22.
18. Levine, P. H. (1988). Factor VIIIC purified from plasma via monoclonal antibodies: human studies. *Seminars in Haematology*, **25**, 38–41.
19. Wood, W. I., Capon, D. J., Simonsen, C. C. (1984). Expression of active human Factor VIII from recombinant DNA clones. *Nature*, **312**, 330–7.
20. White, G. C. (1989). The use of recombinant antihaemophilic factor in the treatment of two patients with classic haemophilia. *New England Journal of Medicine*, **320**, 166–70.
21. Ludlam, C. (1984). Abnormalities of circulating lymphocyte sub-sets in haemophiliacs in an AIDS free population. *Lancet*, **i**, 1431–34.

22. Ragni, M. B., Hanley, E. N. (1989). Septic arthritis in haemophilic patients and infection with human immunodeficiency virus. *Annals of Internal Medicine*, **110(2)**, 168–9.
23. Darby, S. C., Rizza, C. R., Doll, R. (1989). Incidence of AIDS and excessive mortality associated with HIV in haemophiliacs in the United Kingdom. *British Medical Journal*, **298**, 1064–74.
24. MMWR (1987). HIV infection and pregnancies in sexual partners of HIV seropositive haemophiliac men. *Morbidity and Mortality Weekly Report*, **36**, 593–95.

Further reading

Bloom, A. L. and Thomas, D. P. (1987). *Haemostasis and Thrombosis*, Churchill Livingstone, Edinburgh.
Coleman, R. (1987). *Haemostasis and Thrombosis – Basic Principles in Clinical Practice*, Lippincott, Philadelphia.
Jones, P. (1991). *Living with Haemophilia*, 3rd edition, MTP Press Ltd, Lancaster.
Hilgartner, M. W., Pochedly, C. (1989). *Haemophilia in the Child and Adult*, Raven Press Ltd, New York.

4 Part 2 Nursing care of children with haemophilia and HIV infection

Alex Susman-Shaw

Sharing care with other health care agencies

It is important to appreciate the multi-disciplinary nature of care that all children with haemophilia and related coagulation disorders receive. The team-work approach varies in registered Haemophilia Centres throughout the country; some Centres cater solely for children, whilst others provide treatment for children and adults.

Hospital liaison and haemophilia

Each Haemophilia Centre may enlist the skills of the hospital specialist services including the following:

Department of Orthopaedics
General and Paediatric Surgeons
Ear, nose and throat Consultants
Department of Psychology
Department of Genetics
Physiotherapists
Dental services
Dieticians
Department of Social Work
X-ray department
Department of Pathology

There is also liaison with the Community Care Team, providing a comprehensive umbrella of care[1].

Community liaison and haemophilia

The Haemophilia Centre's link with the community is important. The parents of those boys who are infected with HIV may wish to care for them at home, and are encouraged to do so. The family will require help from people in whom they have confidence and who understand the problems of haemophilia and HIV infection. This support and care will come initially from the nursing team working in the Centre, but a time will arise when those nurses will need help from the Community Team. The general practitioner is involved in the child's care throughout his life and his or her help and involvement is invaluable, especially the support that he or she and the Primary Care Team may offer during the terminal stages of the syndrome. There are other knowledgeable and supportive carers in the community from whom the Haemophilia Centre can elist help, for example, voluntary agencies, AIDS Help-lines and AIDS Co-ordinators, together with the extended family, friends and neighbours, where appropriate. However the important need for confidentiality should be remembered and the family's consent for referral should always be gained in the first instance. (See also Chapter 3.)

The haemophilia centre and continuity of care

Co-ordination of the Haemophilia Centre is often managed by the clinical nurse specialist or haemophilia nursing sister, together with the Medical Centre's Director. The doctor has ultimate control and responsibility for all patients with haemophilia. Multidisciplinary clinics are held frequently throughout the year for all children with haemophilia and related disorders, and play an important part in the continuity of care. These relate to both the physical and psychological issues that may affect the child and his family.

The skills of the team are based on accurate and current knowledge of haemophilia and its complications, together with familiarity of the many issues surrounding HIV and AIDS. It is prudent to mention that all carers of children with bleeding disorders, who also may have HIV infection, should not lose themselves in the convoluted problems that encompass HIV. The underlying basic problem of haemophilia may become overlooked and therefore carers should maintain a consistent and non-fragmented approach towards this group of people.

The role of the haemophilia nurse

There is no set description of this role and each Centre may provide a slightly differing working environment. The nurse may become the link person, a clinical practitioner, a teacher (of both families and health care workers), and a friend to his or her patients with listening and counselling as part of the role.

The haemophilia nurse may have been present when the bleeding disorder was initially diagnosed in the child/family and strong relationships will have been established. They have inevitably become increasingly more involved as the advent of HIV infection became apparent in some of this patient population. There is little data to show how best the health care worker can approach this work which is enormously demanding[2] but, because of the evolution of a trusting relationship throughout the years, both children and their families are able to relate to the nurse when problems occur.

Haemophilia is a subtle and disruptive condition which, in spite of treatment for individual bleeding episodes, can still be life-threatening and disabling, both physically and psychologically. There is a risk of iatrogenic infections with blood-borne organisms and the additional knowledge places an enormous emotional burden on patients and their families. (See Chapter 4, Part 1.) Nurses can imagine how parents may feel; many may have become bitter and angry. This stress can be transmitted to their children and families need time to release their anger and talk about their feelings. Nurses may help by offering time and space for families to express their distress. The telephone in the Centre may be in constant use, with the nurse listening, explaining and giving information. Parents may not want set appointments for counselling sessions (although this facility should be available, if appropriate). The time that they need help and support may not be in clinic hours, so health care workers should be able and prepared to work flexible hours in order to meet the needs of these families.

Caring for boys with haemophilia and HIV, together with their families, may also manifest many stress factors amongst professional carers. In order to cope, they need the support of their colleagues and managers, and to be given time to express their own feelings and reflect on their clinical practice.[5] It is becoming generally accepted that no one person alone can support and help a family with HIV. A team-work approach is beneficial for both carer and his family. (See also Chapter 11.)

Home treatment and haemophilia

The availability of treatment of bleeding episodes at home has revolutionised the lives of families living with haemophilia. Instead of numerous hospital visits for treatment, the child can receive infusions of Factor VIII or IX concentrate at home, at school or at work.

This should be given at an early stage of the bleed when treatment is much more effective. This early intervention results in less damage to joints and muscles, thus reducing absences from school or work. Many children who are severely affected by haemophilia are on a home treatment programme. This incorporates teaching and training parents (or other family members) as well as the patient, if appropriate, in the delivery of safe treatment to the child via an intravenous route. The programme includes the following:

- information about bleeding
- instruction about venepuncture
- selection of veins
- use of treatment packs
- storage and disposal of equipment
- record-keeping
- information about replacement Factors
- information about actual infusion[4,5,6].

Each Haemophilia Centre may have a slightly differing approach, but each has similar fundamental objectives of treatment and care. The nurse is involved in the monitoring of home treatment programmes, providing support and continuity of this care.

Children may begin this training for home treatment with their parents when they are five or six years old. However there is no obligation for parents or children to enter the programme if any family member is reluctant or unable to do so. The period of training time varies between families and may depend on motivation, skill and a general attitude of acceptance. In the author's experience all parents are capable of giving a bolus intravenous infusion of replacement therapy providing they are taught correctly and follow set guidelines and procedures. Many children are on self-treatment by the time they reach adolescence.

Where there is a family with one or more members infected by HIV, the nurse has the responsibility of ensuring the family are acquainted with appropriate infectious control precautions. This opportunity to give support and provide a continuity of care may help to alleviate some of the isolation felt by many families with and without HIV infection.

Some factors of influence in haemophilia treatment

When HIV infection became a feature in treatment many parents were reluctant to treat their children with replacement factors. This was partly due to the press and media coverage of HIV and AIDS linked with blood and blood products. There was much uncertainty both medically and socially about the risks of HIV infection. The same reluctance was evident in adults with haemophilia. Parents needed encouragement to treat a bleeding episode rather than to leave it untreated; they became wary of using Factors VIII and IX due to suspicion that re-infection might occur. Medical and nursing staff spend much time reassuring patients, in order that treatment might be continued and quality of life could be maintained and subsequently improved. In the author's experience it has taken a long time for families to understand and believe that the treatment is safe. Regardless of the child's HIV status, all bleeding episodes requiring Factors VIII or IX should be treated.

Considerations for nurses caring for families with haemophilia

Children born into families with a previous history of haemophilia may present the immediate family with concern and anxiety. With a 30 per cent mutation rate in haemophilia, knowledge that their child has the disorder may present enormous distress to parents who have no previous family history of haemophilia. The diagnosis of any abnormality is always traumatic and the anxiety level of parents with haemophilia is high. The further knowledge that they may have to contend with the complexities of HIV-related illness has compounded this already difficult situation. Fear and uncertainty about the future presents yet more anxiety; the nurse may be able to encourage the families to rediscover ways of coping. It will be important for the family to retain independence and confidence in their ability to cope as much as possible.

The obvious bruising in young children is forever present and insinuations of child abuse and non-accidental injury, which may be directed towards the parents and/or family, causes much distress. The health visitor, with help and advice from the Haemophilia Centre nurse, is able to help these families live and cope with the manifestations of haemophilia, and, where necessary, HIV.

Parents have to adjust to having a disrupted family life, caused by numerous hospital visits and the need for urgent treatment. Parents, especially mothers, may feel guilty[7]. Frequent clinic attendances to review HIV positive boys remain an essential part of care.

All nurses working with families with haemophilia and HIV will need to be aware of the many issues surrounding this 'double-edged' problem. Co-ordination of care, anticipation of their needs and a continual updating of information, for both health care workers and the families involved, are all within the haemophilia nurses' sphere of responsibility.

Children with haemophilia and HIV in hospital

These children who are either asymptomatic or symptomatic are nursed with the same degree of care as afforded to any other child (see Chapters 5, 7, 8 and 11). Children who are HIV positive in the ward setting give the staff opportunity to examine hygiene and health education practices[8]. Boys with haemophilia may require surgical procedures such as tonsillectomy and adenoidectomy, orchidopexy, herniotomy, or appendicectomy etc. Boys who are HIV positive should not be excluded from surgery. Medical and nursing staff involved in the care of the child, and *who need to know* of the boy's HIV positive status, should be told. (See Chapter 5.) Any issues arising from the child having haemophilia should be highlighted and forward planning for potential post-operative complications can be anticipated and considered.

Planning and preparation may include the following:

- Reducing any specific equipment and instructions that may identify the child's HIV status to other people on the ward.
- Provision of privacy for parents and child where appropriate.
- Encouragement of staff in participation of HIV and AIDS education and training where necessary.
- Provision of a side room for a child with HIV may be necessary for reasons explained in Chapter 12. However, all health care workers should encourage the child to be part of the open paediatric ward and its activities wherever possible, unless there is a risk of cross infection both to and from the immune compromised child.

Issues for families with children who have differing HIV status

There are several ways a family with haemophilia may be affected by HIV infection.

- Children in families with one or both parents who have HIV infection.
- Boys with siblings with haemophilia some (or one) with HIV, and others unaffected.
- Sisters of boys with haemophilia with and without HIV infection.
- Uncles, nephews and cousins affected by haemophilia and possibly HIV.

Each family unit will have differing physical, emotional and social requirements. The Haemophilia Centre staff will plan and provide care to meet these varying needs. It may be important to remember that many children dislike being 'different' and gentle, simple explanations may help to alleviate some of the anxiety.

There are young people with haemophilia and HIV infection placed in local authority care; their different needs require identification and appropriate support and care can then be implemented.

Haemophilia, HIV and the older child

It would be helpful to find reading material that boys of different ages will understand. To find suitable, comprehensive books and leaflets is no easy task. Parents of boys with haemophilia and HIV should be included in discussions when such books and other reading material may be introduced. It is always important for their hopes and fears to be heard, understood and explored. Leaflets and other reading material are a poor substitute for one-to-one discussion and support. However, the timing has to be right. There may be a strong case for the child's denial. He has a right to this defence; it may be his best way of coping (see Chapter 11).

Issues for families with haemophiliac children who are HIV-negative

Parents of boys who remain HIV negative have said that they feel guilty, and query why their sons remain free of infection when others are not. Some of these parents have sons who are in the same age group as those who are infected, and some have children who were born after heat treatment of replacement factors was introduced.

Parents of many of these boys have told their children of their negative HIV status. The boys are still tested regularly for viral infections, and most children with haemophilia are offered Hepatitis B vaccine. These boys need to be educated in the ways that HIV is spread as do all young people of a similar and appropriate age; they are just as susceptible as any other member of the population.

Unfortunately, due to mass media coverage and ignorance, haemophilia has become synonymous with HIV infection, resulting in many families feeling stigmatised. For many, haemophilia is not divulged to others, especially employers. Those who suffer from haemophilia have become a 'labelled' group and many feel that they cannot blend like others within the community.

Group support for families with haemophilia and HIV infection

There is a variety of support available to families, organised in different ways. Self-help groups, social functions and events especially for children may play a part in helping those to cope with the stress of living with HIV.

In the author's experience, although parents of children with haemophilia and HIV infection are extremely worried and need support, they have not felt it necessary to form a separate support group. Many have not wanted such a group, they do not want to become involved in the problems of others. The local Haemophilia Society group gives all families support, help, counselling and friendship, together with support from the Centre staff.

However, in other areas of the United Kingdom there are groups run by and for parents of children with haemophilia and HIV infection. These have been mutually supportive, especially at times of extra stress when children have become seriously ill and death has occurred.

It is important to note that some families with haemophilia and HIV infection have been reluctant to use the facilities of other agencies catering for the needs of the others with HIV infection and AIDS.

Parents who have chosen not to tell their sons of their HIV status

Coping with the problem of HIV for those parents who have not told their sons of their HIV status may present difficulties for the families and health care workers. If the boys are well and remaining asymptomatic their parents may feel lulled into a false sense of security, thinking and believing that 'nothing may happen'; this is a coping strategy and should be acknowledged as such.

Many Haemophilia Centre staff have known parents who have hidden the condition from their sons. Parents turn off television sets, hide newspapers and cut out relevant articles in order to protect their children from learning about HIV infection associated with haemophilia. Because parent's anxiety levels are so high and they trust the staff so implicitly, the health care workers have felt and still feel their 'hands are tied'. Many parents try to keep the diagnosis entirely to themselves, not even telling other family members and relatives[9]. (See also Chapter 4, Part 1.)

The role of the haemophilia nurse in schools

Continuity of care extends to the child in school. Here the haemophilia nurse has the role of an educator. Because haemophilia is frightening to many, and contact with sufferers is rare, teachers may be worried and uneasy about accepting a child with the disorder. The nurse can visit schools, providing support to the staff, giving information, dispelling myths and providing a contact. Rather than having an impersonal hospital for referral, this tangible link gives the school staff a feeling of security, particularly as school visits can be flexible.

There is still a general lack of understanding in the general public about HIV infection and AIDS; school visits are one way of disseminating the information. Children with haemophilia have been chided by their peer groups. Cruelty amongst children is not unknown. Many boys with haemophilia have been subjected to unnecessary suffering and have been shunned at school because haemophilia is associated with HIV infection. Teachers have been frightened of dealing with an injured child who has a bleeding disorder. The nurse helps by giving information to groups at school and providing specific literature. She can also advise on types of sport and exercise – those which are beneficial and those which are harmful – thus encouraging the child to integrate as normally as possible without too many unnecessary restrictions. The school nurse will also need to be briefed on the problems and treatment of haemophilia so that she is able to help and support the boys[10]. The safety of blood products and venepuncture equipment on school premises is of paramount importance. Arrangements for boys to treat themselves with Factor replacement at school are made with the education authorities. They recognise the effectiveness and benefits of immediate treatment with resulting reduction of lost school hours due to this early intervention.

Information given to young people about coping with bleeding and injuries

Children with haemophilia are advised to wear identity bracelets or necklaces. All those who are registered as having a bleeding disorder are issued with a special 'green card' which should contain relevant information about their condition. The older boy may well know about the dangers of blood contamination because of the problems of hepatitis. It is suggested that mouth bleeds are stemmed by the use of a topical medication supplied by the Haemophilia Centre, and applied with a small dressing using finger pressure. Nose bleeds are treated by sitting the child upright with his head leaning forward and pressure applied on the upper half of the nose. If bleeding continues for any length of time then Factor replacement, together with medical advice, should be sought. Where necessary, it may be prudent to reinforce the need for appropriate care to be taken when there is blood spillage from *any* member of the community. This will lessen the risk of cross infection and identification of a person with HIV infection. (See also Chapter 8, Part 2 and Chapter 12.)

Health education and haemophilia

Older boys become very concerned and anxious about how HIV will affect their relationships. Many adolescents find it difficult to talk to their parents, so they may come to the centre to talk to someone they know well, who they trust to give them accurate and helpful information. It has been stated that there are not many nurses who can talk about sexual issues and problems with adolescents[11]. These young men feel very responsible and do not want to pass on any infection. A number of them may abstain from having relationships because of the difficulties that may arise around sexual issues. They may also be in a quandary – should they tell their girlfriends that they are infected with HIV? Should they tell their girlfriends that they have haemophilia? All adolescents attending the centre are given advice and encouraged to practice safer sex; this information is given to the appropriate age group.

Conclusion

Families with haemophilia and HIV infection have two life threatening disorders to contend with simultaneously. The physical, emotional and social needs of the families challenge all aspects of health care, and a team approach is essential. Inevitably, the haemophilia nurse will be closely involved and his or her work will affect the quality of care that people with haemophilia and HIV receives.

References

1. Sharp, P. *et al.* (1989). Nursing care of HIV positive patients. *Health Care Management*, **4**, 2.
2. Claxton, R. (1989). Looking after the children. *Nursing Times*, **85(39)**, 41–3.
3. Weller, B. (1989). Children and HIV infection. *Nursing Standard*, **4**, 11th Oct., 50–2.
4. Susman-Shaw, A. (1981). Home treatment for children with haemophilia. *Nursing Times*, **77(39)**, 1656–60.
5. Jones, P. *et al.* (1978). A home therapy in the United Kingdom, 1975–1976. *British Medical Journal*, **1(6125)**, 1447–50.
6. Ingram, G. I. C. *et al.* (1979). Home treatment in haemophilia, clinical, social and economic advantages. *Clinical Lab. Haematology*, **1**, 13–27.
7. Gregory, M., Foy, F. (1988). The anxiety factor. Spotlight on children. *Nursing Times*, **84**, 20th Apr., 71–2.
8. Macqueen, S. (1989). Positive practice. Spotlight on children. *Nursing Times*, **85(43)**, 67–8.
9. Anonymous. Young haemophiliacs not told of HIV. *Nursing Times*, **84**, 38.
10. Sadler, C. (1988). AIDS in schools. *Nursing Times*, **84**, 16–17.
11. Thompson, J. (1990). Sexuality: the adolescent and cancer. *Nursing Standard*, **4**, 37.26–8.

Further reading

Aronstam, A. (1985). *Haemophilic Bleeding*, Bailliere Tindall, London.

Berger, M. (1989). *Understanding Haemophilia*, Ashgrove Press, Bath.

Darby, S. C. *et al.* (1989). Incidence of AIDS and excess of mortality with HIV in haemophiliacs in the United Kingdom: A report on behalf of the Directors of the Haemophilia Centres in the United Kingdom. *British Medical Journal*, **298**, 1064–5.

Esiri, M. M. *et al.* (1989). Neuropathology of HIV infection in haemophiliacs. Comparative necropsy study. *British Medical Journal*, **299**, 1312–15.

Jones, J. (1990). A question of empathy. *Nursing Times*, **86**, 2.

Jones, P. (1991). *Living With Haemophilia*, 3rd edition, MTP Press, Lancaster.

Meerstadt, T., Brueton, M. J. (1987). Paediatric AIDS. *Maternal and Child Health*, **July**, 218–24.

Turner, T. A. (1988). A helping hand for haemophiliacs. *Nursing Times*, **84**, 49.

Ward Wimmer, D. (1988). Nursing care of children with HIV infection. *Nursing Clinics of North America*, **23**, 4.

5   Legal and ethical issues of paediatric HIV infection

Reg Pyne

Law and ethics

In every situation in which practitioners of medicine, nursing, midwifery and other regulated health professions exercise their judgements and apply their knowledge and skill in the interests of patients and the public, they must operate within a framework of law. Professional practice, however, trans-cends the law. Such practitioners must practice their profession in a manner that will be perceived as ethical by peers in their own and related health professions and by the public. Since this is the case whatever the patient group, it must be so when applied to children.

Some might argue that a chapter which is concerned with legal issues in respect of paediatric HIV infection is unnecessary in a specialist book of this kind, since there are excellent books available which describe and elaborate upon those aspects of the law which apply to the patient with AIDS or who is HIV-positive as much as to any other patient. Such books explain that the HIV-positive patient is entitled to the same protection from the law in respect of consent, confidentiality and professional liability as any other patient. The same applies to their explanation of health and safety law.

My response would be that given that there are a limited number of specific laws and caselaw related to AIDS and HIV infection, and given also that certain aspects of international law take on a greater significance in respect of AIDS and HIV infection than with any other disease, such a chapter is justified. It might also be the case that the more that the relevant national and international law is described and understood, the more it will be accepted by the population as reasonable and protected from those who, out of misunder-standing or prejudice, lobby for it to be changed so far as persons with HIV infection are concerned. As the World Health Organisation has stated:

Personal and public reaction to AIDS throughout the world has been of considerable depth and extent. Fear of AIDS and stigmatisation of different groups (homosexual men, haemophiliacs, injecting drug users and female prostitutes) have become common. Wherever those free from HIV feel threatened by those infected with HIV, especially where the latter form a defined group . . . there may be calls for marking out and isolating those infected. As the toll of clinical disease rises, there will be increasing pressure on the authorities to take further action and adopt approaches that may or may not be effective or have any rational justification[1].

Part of the role of professional practitioners in this specialist area must therefore be to protect the existing law and seek to see it enhanced appropriately. In this context it is worth seeking to learn by reminding ourselves how the problem of syphilis infection was dealt with in the United Kingdom. Between 1864 and 1869 three 'Contagious Diseases Acts' were passed. These authorised the detention of suspected prostitutes in certain garrison towns and ports, statutory medical examination and compulsory treatment while in detention. This scheme was strongly opposed by the medical profession which resented the policing role forced upon it and proved to be of no use. The Acts were repealed in 1886. Eventually in 1916, a Royal Commission on Venereal Diseases recommended the establishment of special clinics offering free treatment on an entirely voluntary basis and guaranteeing complete anonymity and confidentiality. The contention was that this would succeed in minimising spread through early detection for which voluntary co-operation was essential. The recommendation was accepted. The scheme exists to this day and has achieved a high level of success. Surely there is a message there for the advocates of discriminatory legislation.

The relevance of international law

It is worth noting that certain clauses of international law have a relevance to the development of national legislation as it applies to persons with HIV infection. Since 1945, the international community of nations has established a binding code of international human rights. This flows from the United Nations Charter of 1945, the Universal Declaration of Human Rights of 1948 and the two International Covenants (one on Civil and Political Rights, the other on Economic, Social and Cultural Rights) which came into force in 1976. The resultant code declares and protects a range of rights for '. . . everyone, without distinction of any kind, such as race, colour, sex, language, religion, political or other opinion, national or social origin, property, birth or status'. For any right to be effective, a corresponding duty must be imposed on some other person or authority. In the case of human rights the duty falls on the state which is obliged to ensure, to the best of its abilities, that the rights of its inhabitants will be respected. It can therefore be seen that a number of important clauses in international law underpin the resolve of any country or state to ensure that its national laws do not discriminate against persons with a particular infection or illness by introducing irrational and impractical laws.

Legal issues of HIV infection

The legal issues which require specific consideration are a product of both the character of the infection or disease and the reaction it has provoked from a largely uninformed or ill-informed public. They focus primarily around the two important issues of confidentiality and consent.

Confidentiality

This aspect of the subject brings the legal and ethical issues into play together. One of the most fundamental ethical obligations owed by a member of any of the health care professions to his or her patient is to respect all confidential information from or about that patient. The Handbook of Medical Ethics published by the British Medical Association states that 'a doctor must preserve secrecy in all he knows'.[2] The United Kingdom Central Council for

Nursing, Midwifery and Health Visiting (UKCC), in its document 'Confidentiality'[3] advises its practitioners in the following terms:

It is essential that nurses, midwives and health visitors recognise the fundamental right of their patients or clients to information about them being kept private and secure. This point is sharply reinforced by only brief consideration of the personal, social or legal repercussions which might follow unauthorised disclosure of information concerning a person's health or illness.

'Confidentiality' is a rule with certain exceptions. There is no statutory right of confidentiality; but there is also no bar to an aggrieved individual bringing a common law case before a civil court alleging breach of confidentiality and seeking financial recompense.

It is essential that before determining that a particular set of circumstances constitute such an exception, the practitioner must be satisfied that the best interests of the patient/client are served thereby or the wider public interest necessitates disclosure.

This allows for rare and specific exceptions to the general principle of confidentiality and non-disclosure. The justification for any exception is to be found only in the best interests of the patient or in the public interest. It is unlikely that both will be served by the same disclosure. Any practitioner deciding, after due consideration, to breach a confidence exposes himself or herself to action in the courts.

AIDS, confidentiality and the courts

Through one significant case in 1988 the courts have revealed their position in respect of the preservation of confidentiality, in particular where it relates to AIDS. A health authority sought to restrain a national newspaper from publishing information to the effect that two doctors it employed were still practising although they were diagnosed as having AIDS. The information had come to the notice of the newspaper as a result of a breach of confidentiality by another employee of the health authority. For the defendant newspaper it was argued that disclosure was in the public interest and that, even if there had been a breach of confidence, it was justified. In his judgement on the case the judge stated:

Confidentiality is of paramount importance to such patients, including doctors. The plaintiffs take care to ensure it. Their servants are contractually bound to respect it. If it is breached, or if the patients have grounds for thinking that it may be or has been breached, they will be reluctant to come forward for and to continue with treatment and counselling. If the actual or apprehended breach is to the press that reluctance is likely to be very great[4].

In that case the judge rejected the arguments of the newspaper and found for the health authority. That does not alter the fact, however, that the duty of confidentiality is not absolute. The courts recognise a number of exceptions in the form of situations where the law requires disclosure: where information is required to assist in the investigation or prosecution of what is deemed to be a serious crime, disclosure is judged to prevent a continuing serious threat to the health of other people, or disclosure is believed to be necessary in the public interest. The public interest and health risk justifications are likely to be subjected to strong challenge whenever applied. This is particularly the case in respect of HIV and AIDS because of the extra statutory protection the confidentiality issue has been given.

The relevance of a specific section of law

Although misleadingly termed given certain of its modes of transmission, AIDS is a venereal disease for the purposes of the law. Therefore the National Health Service (Venereal Diseases) Regulations 1974 (as amended) apply. Under these regulations, health authorities (not general practitioners, private hospitals or clinics) are required to take steps to ensure that any information capable of identifying an individual, that is obtained by officers of the authority with respect to any sexually transmitted disease, shall not be disclosed except for the purpose of communicating information to a medical practitioner, a person employed under the direction of a medical practitioner in connection with treatment, or for the purpose of such treatment or prevention. It is generally assumed that, although HIV infection is not transmitted through sexual contact exclusively, these regulations would apply to all HIV cases. Nothing in the regulations would prevent disclosure where the law requires it or the patient/client authorises disclosure.

Inadvertent disclosure to the media

As was illustrated by the action before the courts taken by a health authority (judgement quoted above), certain sections of the press have a tendency to demonstrate a particular interest in the subject of HIV infection and AIDS. Such an interest is as likely to be shown in respect of an infected child as any other patient. It is important, therefore, that nurses be on their guard and mindful of the ease with which confidentiality can be inadvertently breached. To respond to a telephone call from a person who purports to be a relative may result in an unintended release of confidential information. Indeed, there are some circumstances in which even to acknowledge that a named person is a patient on a particular ward or unit can lead to an inference about their diagnosis. Health authority policies should ensure that safe practices exist for the identification of callers and that information is not released to telephone enquirers without the agreement of the patient or parent/guardian. Parents of children with HIV infection or AIDS should be informed about all enquiries received and their wishes as to disclosure respected totally. The same principle must apply in respect of requests for information from the media.

The diagnosis – staff awareness

Another aspect of the confidentiality issue that arises in respect of HIV and AIDS is the question of which members of staff need to know the patient's diagnosis. The very fact that the question arises is an expression of a subliminally held belief that if the patient is HIV positive or has AIDS some additional infection control procedures are required. However, the infection control procedures required for the safe care of *all* patients need to be made known to and observed by *all* categories of staff. In such circumstances the patient's diagnosis can remain confidential to the child patient, the patient's parents/guardians and the professional staff providing direct patient care.

The diagnosis – the patient and the family

Just as a judgement has to be made as to which members of the staff of a hospital or clinic need to know about a patient's diagnosis or HIV status, so a judgement must be made about the sharing of such information with a patient who is a minor and with his or her parents.

In its advisory document *Exercising Accountability*[5], the UKCC states:

If it is to be believed that, on occasions, practitioners withhold information from their patients, the damage to public trust and confidence in the profession, on which the introduction to the Code of Professional Conduct places great emphasis, will be enormous.

This is yet another area in which judgements have to be made and introduces another facet of the exercise of accountability. If it is accepted that the patient has a right to information about his condition, it follows that the professional practitioners involved in his care have a duty to provide such information. Recognition of the patient's condition and the likely effect of the information might lead the professionals to be selective about 'what' and 'when' but the responsibility is on them to provide information. There may be occasions on which, after consultation with the relatives of a patient by the health professionals involved in that patient's care, some information is temporarily withheld. If, however, something less than the whole truth is told at a particular point in time it should never be because the practitioner is unable to cope with the effects of telling the whole truth. Such controlled release of information (i.e. less than the whole truth) should only ever be in the interests of the patient, and the practitioner should be able to justify the action taken.

I cannot emphasise the contents of that quotation too strongly.

As with other aspects of paediatric nursing, the parents will require support throughout the illness of their child. Where the child proves to be HIV positive, it may be that the mother is herself infected. The normal anxieties of a concerned parent may therefore be compounded by guilt, presenting an additional problem for the professional carers. In such cases, the legal principle that must be applied is that of what needs to be done to satisfy the duty of care owed to the patient, the family and to society. On to that must be superimposed the ethical burden of telling the truth only to those who need to know and concealing confidential information from others. The case for immediate honesty with the parents and with the child at the earliest possible stage seems self-evident.

The status of minors

Exploration of a range of issues related to confidentiality inevitably links to some aspects of consent and makes it necessary to comment briefly upon the status of those persons we know as minors. Paediatric nurses, since they care for minors (i.e. persons under the age of 18 years) should be knowledgeable about a number of special provisions.

From the age of 18 years, adults are able to make their own decisions about their medical care, provided they are mentally competent. This extends to participation in research, whether of a therapeutic nature or otherwise. For those who have not attained the age of 18 years the situation is somewhat different.

Under the terms of Section 8 of the Family Law Reform Act (1969) a minor of 16 or 17 years of age can give a valid consent to treatment. That authority does not extend to participation in any research programme.

The power given to a minor of 16 or 17 years of age to consent to treatment has not affected a parent's right to give consent. Clashes of view seem unlikely but have been known to occur. In a situation where the parents and their 17-year-old child disagree about a form of treatment, the parallel nature of these powers might become a matter for consideration by the courts.

The situation is different in respect of children under 16 years of age, but far from absolute. While the parents or guardians are able to give consent for treatment, if the minor is deemed by his or her professional carers to be mature and capable of understanding, he or she can give a valid consent to treatment or withhold such consent. In *Law, Ethics and Medicine*[6], Skegg states that:

The view that at common law all minors are incapable of consenting to medical procedures results from a fundamental misconception of such procedures in relation to the criminal and civil law.

This may come to have, by analogy, significant implications in the field of HIV infection and AIDS. [See also the Children Act, 1989. Ed.]

The sexually active HIV-positive minor

One such implication may arise when a minor – possibly below the age of 16 years – is found to be HIV positive and it is apparent that he or she is sexually active. The case for ensuring that the minor is told of his or her HIV status is self-evident. It is obvious that the information needs to be accompanied by expert counselling and guidance about sexual practices. It would also seem wise to urge that the parents or guardians be told so as to assist through what is going to be a difficult period for the infected individual and the family.

What is to be done, however, when the infected minor appears to understand his or her condition, seems to understand the risk posed by unprotected intercourse with others, but appears not to care, has no intention of telling the diagnosis to parents/guardians and presses the medical and nursing staff not to breach confidentiality on the issue?

The situation has some similarity to the case heard by the House of Lords in 1985 (Gillick v West Norfolk and Wisbech Area Health Authority and the Department of Health and Social Security)[7] when the Lords decided that, in exceptional circumstances, a doctor could provide contraceptive advice and treatment to a girl under 16 years without the parents' consent. The similarity has its limits, however, since in that case it could be argued that the best interests of a minor known to be sexually active were the prime consideration. In the case of the sexually active minor who is HIV positive the wider public interest is a factor which cannot be ignored. Refusal to comply with the request not to disclose to parent/guardian, while it may not eventually prove beneficial, would appear justifiable as satisfying the principles of the law with regard to both the 'best interests' of others and 'duty of care' to others.

Parents/guardians

Just as parents/guardians need both short term and continuing help in that situation, so do they where their HIV-positive child has learning difficulties or has a tendency to bite other people. Each of these situations emphasises the importance of matters which are not the subject of this chapter (modes of transmission, control of infection measures). They also emphasise, yet again, that the ethical burdens borne by nurses include those of ensuring that they are well informed, and consequently ensuring that they play their full part in public education and the rejection of dangerous mythology. The responsibility of the nurse certainly extends to discussing with a parent/guardian the true nature of the disease, its modes of transmission and risks, and in every way assisting him/her to arrive at informed decisions about the relevant 'other people' who need to be told of the HIV status of a particular child. The difficulties in this respect cannot be overestimated. On occasions the nurse may even encounter one parent who is reluctant to or even refuses to share information that he or she finds distasteful with the other parent. Once again, whether viewed from a legal or ethical perspective, the 'best interests' and 'duty of care' principles have to be applied by the practitioner in deciding whether to inform the second parent or partner.

Injecting drug users in hospital

Some persons classified as minors who are admitted to a hospital or attending its clinics may have become infected through their habit of intravenous drug use and the sharing of equipment. It may even be that such minors are engaging in their habit while on hospital premises and that the drugs used cannot have been obtained legally.

This can raise very severe difficulties for the practitioners concerned. On the one hand they have knowledge of drugs being illegally obtained, possessed and used. On the other hand they know that to involve the police at that particular stage may well destroy a developing therapeutic relationship. The result may be that the individual does not amend his or her sexual practices and start to behave more responsibly, thus proving a danger to other people, and persists with the abuse of drugs. The dilemma this can cause for caring individual practitioners is enormous. The judgement to be made is difficult.

Anonymous HIV testing

In November 1988, the Secretary of State for Health (Kenneth Clarke) announced new steps to monitor the spread of HIV infection[8]. One of these steps was to be the development of methods of obtaining better epidemiological data by a system of anonymous testing of residual blood for HIV antibodies after the prescribed tests had been completed. It was stated that the Government saw no legal or ethical objection to such testing. The Medical Research Council was required to bring forward proposals for the programme of anonymous screening within three months.

When the resultant proposals became available for perusal in 1989, they faced a certain amount of challenge. Not everyone held the Government's opinion that there was no legal or ethical objection to such an anonymous prevalence testing programme. It was initially to involve specimens of blood taken from patients attending a substantial number of genito-urinary medicine clinics and antenatal clinics, and was to be extended to include a wide range of in-patients and out-patients at general hospitals, and eventually to phenylketonuria test samples from neonates.

Indeed, although it was said that there were no legal objections to anonymous testing, it was not possible to locate any published statement supporting this view. Articles stating the opposite point of view were, however, to be found. For example, in the Law Society's *Gazette* of 15 January 1989 and 1 March 1989 there appeared two articles written jointly by Ian Kennedy (Professor of Medical Law and Ethics, Kings College, London) and Andrew Grubb (Law Fellow, Fitzwilliam College, Cambridge)[9,10]. In the first of these articles the authors state[9]:

The legality of testing without consent is obviously important. The issue is not, however, only a matter of law. There are ethical considerations which transcend the law. . . . That which is lawful may be unethical.

In the second article[10] the authors specifically addressed the subject of anonymous testing:

Dr X takes blood with A's consent to test it for specified purposes. Unknown to A, Dr X intends to test it also for HIV infection, and intends to do so in circumstances in which the identity of the donor of the blood sample cannot be known (i.e. one form of 'anonymised testing').

. . . Here the doctor has removed that which will identify the patient before sending it for testing. This is one of the situations which raise the issue of what has become known as 'anonymised testing'.

Does the removal of the identifying features make the doctor's conduct lawful, since otherwise we have seen that the conduct amounts to both a battery and a breach of duty in negligence?

Undoubtedly, the doctor's conduct compounds the illegality in that he is exposed to further liability in negligence. This is because the doctor has placed himself in a position whereby he is incapable of carrying out his duty of care to the patient. If the test proves positive, the doctor will not be able to identify which patient he must care for. In effect, this amounts to an abandonment of his patient. Furthermore, in evaluating the doctor's conduct, a court would not ignore the fact that the doctor is depriving the patient of the information necessary to allow him the opportunity to behave responsibly and thereby the doctor may also be jeopardising society at large.

After long and careful deliberation, and only after achieving certain improvements it saw as essential, the United Kingdom Central Council for Nursing, Midwifery and Health Visiting indicated its support for the anonymous testing programme on utilitarian grounds, provided that a list of key principles could be satisfied. These are stated in the UKCC's circular PC/89/01[11].

A specific research protocol for each test group must have been approved by the local ethical committee of the health authority from which the blood specimens are to be obtained prior to the commencement of any unlinked anonymous test programme;

the health authority, as an associated part of the research approval, must have considered and acted upon any resource implications for its professional staff and pronounced itself satisfied;

prior to the commencement of any such approved research programme, those whose blood may be used for unlinked anonymous screening have been able to become aware of the monitoring programme (through a general public information campaign supplemented by easily understood posters and leaflets made available in locations where blood will be taken and in the full range of languages appropriate to the known patient/client population) and of their right to state that their blood should not be used for this purpose;

all registered nurses, midwives and health visitors employed in places from which samples are being obtained for this prevalence testing programme must be made aware of that fact in order:

that they may answer honestly any questions put to them by patients and clients about the full range of purposes for which blood samples will or may be tested, and they may consider how best to act to protect the interests of any patients or clients whose transient or permanent condition results in an inability to consider and/or understand the available information literature.

there must be no possible detriment to those whose blood is or is not screened as part of their unlinked anonymous HIV screening programmes; any patient or client who objects to participation in the test programme should have his or her wishes respected fully and should not: be discriminated against in any way; or be identified as being higher risk than those who have not objected and have required treatment withheld or suffer any other detriment.

the amount of blood taken on any occasion should be only that which would normally be taken for the specific tests ordered by the patient's medical practitioner.

The testing of phenylketonuria test samples within this prevalence testing programme raises additional questions, since the baby is being used as a surrogate to assess the HIV status of the mother at the time of delivery.

Bearing in mind the strident arguments which can be heard urging anonymous testing in a variety of other circumstances, none of which appear supportable on practical grounds, this anonymous prevalence testing programme must be studied with great care. In the ultimate, its justification can only lie in the provision of resources sufficient to meet established need in future years.

Funding and managing care

At present the occurrence of the disease in children will have been more a product of the transfusion of infected blood or blood products than other causes; however, this will change. More children of infected mothers will be found to be seropositive in their own right beyond 18 months of age. Some minors may have become infected as a result of injecting drug use with shared and contaminated equipment, or of sexual abuse.

It is important that, as advocates for the larger number of children who will undoubtedly present with the infection and with clinical disease in the future, health professionals seek to maintain the Government's level of awareness about the nature, size and cost of providing care to this group of patients and support for their families. It is also incumbent on them to monitor the development of the NHS purchaser-provider contract arrangements and to ensure that this particular vulnerable and dependent group (for which special funding has been made available to the present) are provided for in a satisfactory way.

Drug trials and associated issues

The incurable nature of the disease renders those suffering from it more exposed than the average patient to approaches that they (or their parents or guardians on their behalf) might consent either to an agreement that a new drug (which might delay the progress of the disease or relieve some of its symptoms) might be tried, or that a known drug might be administered by a route that is not within the product licence.

Where either of these situations arises, bearing in mind the natural tendency of the patient with an incurable condition to clutch at anything which offers the slightest hope, it is essential that the patient or parent/guardian is informed fully about the proposal and able to make a considered decision. It would not be acceptable, for example, for a medication to be administered to a child by a method or in a quantity that fell outside the product licence without consulting the parents/guardians and obtaining their agreement. Where the child is of sufficient maturity to participate in the decision-making they should be consulted.

The HIV-positive health care worker

Contrary to the general assumption, professional practitioners with HIV infection or its consequent clinical illness are more at risk of opportunistic infections from their patients than the patients are at risk from their practitioners.

This matter and a range of related issues are faced squarely by the UKCC in its statement *AIDS and HIV Infection*, the current edition of which was issued in 1989[12]. It raises a number of points which are essential to any consideration of the legal and ethical issues of HIV infection.

Resuscitation and AIDS

An ethical dilemma for discussion

A 14-year-old boy is in your ward, gravely ill with AIDS, the result of a transfusion of infected blood used in the treatment of his haemophiliac condition. The clinical disease has been manifested over a period of time to the great distress of the boy's mother and elder sister. The boy is wasted and is experiencing both distress and pain. It seems clear that he will die within a matter of days. This information is given by a junior doctor to the parents in the presence of the ward sister. The boy's mother is entirely accepting of the situation and indicates that death will be a relief and a release for all of them. She adds that this same view had been expressed by her intelligent son a few weeks before. The ward sister knows this to be true, for it occurred in her presence and in a discussion in which she participated. The mother indicates that she wants his dying moments to be as peaceful as possible and requires no attempts to resuscitate him.

She is taken aback when the boy's father, who had not been party to the discussion and had not seen his son frequently due to travelling in the course of his business, disagrees strongly. He argues that while there is life there is hope for a cure, and that it is the doctor's sacred duty to seek to sustain life at all times, irrespective of the disease, its poor prognosis, or the fact that no means of cure appears to be in sight.

In the face of this firmly stated view the doctor seeks to discuss the situation but is told by the father there is nothing to discuss since his mind is made up. The mother breaks down and cries in great distress. The ward sister knows the father's decision to be a betrayal of his son's wishes.

What should the ward sister do or say? What do you think you would do in these circumstances?

Education and ethical responsibility

In his closing address to the joint UK Health Departments and Health Education Authority Symposium 'HIV and AIDS – An assessment of current and future spread in the UK', held on 24 November 1989, Sir Donald Maitland (Chairman of the Health Education Authority) said:

Information and education remain the most effective means of preventing the spread of HIV infection. We need to sustain and develop our health education work.

In addition, the joint Chairman of the Symposium, Mrs Virginia Bottomley (Minister of State for Health) stated:

No one can afford the luxury of complacency or cynicism and neither should we be deceived into believing that HIV and AIDS are not issues for the population as a whole. To do so would frankly be to fail in our responsibility to future generations[13].

Conclusion

At the beginning of this chapter I stated that professional practice transcends the law. In doing so it carries us into consideration not only of what is lawful but what is ethical. In conclusion, I contend that to behave ethically, nurses must be informed about HIV infection and AIDS, must play their full part in educating the public, and must strive to destroy the dangerous mythology that only serves to isolate all those unfortunate enough to be afflicted with HIV infection.

References

1. World Health Organisation (1988). *Guidelines for the Development of a National AIDS Prevention and Control Programme*, WHO, Geneva.
2. British Medical Association (1988). *Philosophy and Practice of Medical Ethics*, BMA, London.
3. United Kingdom Central Council for Nursing, Midwifery and Health Visiting (1987). *Confidentiality. An Elaboration of Clause 9 of the Second Edition of the UKCC's Code of Professional Conduct for the Nurse, Midwife and Health Visitor*, UKCC, London.
4. Second Volume, *All England Law Reports* (1988), X v Y.
5. United Kingdom Central Council for Nursing, Midwifery and Health Visiting (1989). *Exercising Accountability. A framework to assist nurses, midwives and health visitors to consider ethical aspects of professional practice*, UKCC, London.
6. Skegg, P. D. G. (1985). *Law Ethics and Medicine*, Clarendon Press, London.
7. Third Volume, *All England Law Reports* (1985). Gillick v West Norfolk and Wisbech Area Health Authority and the Department of Health and Social Security.
8. Department of Health (1988). Press Release – *Government announces new steps to monitor the spread of HIV infection*. DOH, London.
9. Kennedy, I., Grubb, A. (1989). Testing for HIV Infection, the legal framework. *The Law Society's Gazette*, **7**.
10. Kennedy, I., Grubb, A. (1989). Testing for HIV Infection: further examples. *The Law Society's Gazette*, **8**.
11. United Kingdom Central Council for Nursing, Midwifery and Health Visiting (1989). *Anonymous Testing for the Prevalence of the Human Immunodeficiency Virus (HIV)*. Circular No. PC/89/01. UKCC, London.
12. United Kingdom Central Council for Nursing, Midwifery and Health Visiting (1989). *UKCC Statement on AIDS and HIV Infection*. Circular No. PC/89/02. UKCC, London.
13. UK Health Departments and Health Education Authority. Proceedings of the Symposium held on 24 November 1989.

Further reading

The Children Act (1989). [This Act will be implemented in October 1991. Ed.]

6 Pregnancy, childbirth and HIV infection

Janette Brierley and Carolyn Roth

Introduction

Although the total number of reported cases of Acquired Immune Deficiency Syndrome (AIDS) in children in the UK is currently low[1], the numbers are bound to rise as the incidence of Human Immunodeficiency Virus (HIV) infection amongst women of childbearing age increases. It has been estimated that in New York City 1 in 80 births is to an HIV-infected woman[2,3]. HIV/AIDS is now one of the ten leading causes of death in women of childbearing age in the US, and at the current rate of increase it is expected to become one of the five leading causes by 1991[4].

Most paediatric HIV infection is due to perinatal transmission[5] and the proportion of children infected by contaminated blood and blood products will diminish as the screening of blood becomes universal.

The coexistence of HIV and pregnancy gives rise to innumerable ethical and emotional dilemmas for the pregnant woman and those who provide a maternity service. These issues require careful consideration when planning care of women during pregnancy.

Should women be screened for HIV during pregnancy?

The seriousness of HIV infection, the poor prognosis of the disease and the possibility of transmission to the newborn perinatally, appear to constitute strong grounds for encouraging antenatal testing of pregnant women for HIV. In addition, antenatal care embodies a tradition of screening for the early detection of complications to the woman and/or her unborn child and testing for HIV would seem to fit well into this pattern of care.

However, even in well established antenatal screening programmes, such as amniocentesis for detection of chromosomal abnormality, there are glaring shortcomings. Facilities are often lacking for helping women deal with the need to make complex and difficult decisions on the basis of the critical information discovered by testing[6].

Furthermore, diagnosis of HIV infection will have a negative impact on the life of the pregnant woman which will extend far beyond decision making in relation to pregnancy. Individuals with HIV infection are subjected to enormous social stigma and this cannot be ignored when the issue of testing pregnant women is considered.

If HIV testing is to be made available as part of care during pregnancy, it must be based on an understanding of the needs of the HIV-positive woman.

The service must ensure adequate provision of information, complete protection of confidentiality, counselling and support, so that women are given the opportunity to make a genuinely informed choice about this serious issue.

The significance of HIV for pregnancy

The effect of HIV on pregnancy outcome

Data on the pregnancy outcome in asymptomatic HIV-positive women do not suggest that HIV infection in itself has an adverse effect on the outcome of pregnancy.

An Edinburgh study looked at the outcome of pregnancy in a group of HIV-infected women all of whom were injecting drug users or partners of drug users. They tended to be young, unmarried, heavy smokers and to be from deprived areas of the city. When compared with a group of HIV-negative women from the same background there were no differences in maternal pregnancy complications, mean birthweight, gestational age at delivery, perinatal mortality or fetal abnormality. There was a higher rate of spontaneous abortion in the HIV-positive women. However both groups of women had rates of premature delivery and intrauterine growth retardation almost three times higher, and low birthweight almost four times higher, than in the total Edinburgh City population. The results suggest that drug use rather than HIV positivity accounted for the poor fetal outcome[7].

A similar study in New York of women in a methadone programme showed no differences in the frequency of spontaneous or elective abortion, ectopic pregnancy, preterm delivery, stillbirth or low birthweight between HIV-positive and HIV-negative women[8].

However, a study in Zaire of the perinatal outcome of infants born to HIV-positive women compared with a similar group of babies whose mothers were HIV-negative demonstrated increased rates of prematurity, low birthweight and a higher rate of neonatal death. Of the HIV-positive mothers, 18 per cent had AIDS[9]. These adverse outcomes may be linked to the high proportion of immune compromised HIV-positive mothers. It is probable that many of the neonatal deaths were associated with low birthweight and prematurity, rather than a direct effect of HIV infection on the baby.

The risk of pregnancy for the mother

There are theoretical grounds for a concern that pregnancy combined with HIV infection might accelerate the course of illness[10]. Studies early in the epidemic suggested that pregnancy increased an HIV-infected woman's risk of developing AIDS[11]. The findings were based on the pregnancies of women who had already delivered a baby which had developed AIDS. In light of subsequent prospective studies, the high rate of illness progression in these women may have reflected their relatively advanced state of illness rather than an effect of pregnancy itself.

A more recent prospective study in New York found no excess progression in HIV-related disease status in pregnant women as compared with non-pregnant counterparts[10]. However, a recent study by Biggar *et al.*[12] suggests that pregnancy may accelerate HIV-induced immune compromise, but the study does not clearly show that pregnancy alone is responsible for this.

Clearly there is a need for further investigation of this question. It is impossible to provide a definitive answer about the effect of pregnancy on HIV disease progression. Many of the women who have been studied are also drug users and this may influence results. Perhaps until further evidence is available, it would be prudent to acknowledge a potential additional risk from pregnancy, but stress that preliminary results of controlled studies have not demonstrated an acceleration of HIV-related disease[10].

The risks of infection for the fetus and newborn

HIV is transplacentally transmitted to the fetus[13]. Theoretically, the fetus may be infected by exposure to blood at delivery, but this is currently impossible to confirm. Infection rates in the newborn vary in different studies, possibly due to differing stages of maternal illness. Initial findings of the European Collaborative Study demonstrated a transmission rate of 24 per cent[14]. More recent findings of this ongoing study suggest that only one in five or six HIV-positive women enrolled transmitted the virus to their babies[15]. However, transmission rates must be viewed with caution given that estimates of the risk vary so widely from study to study and there is still much debate about risk factors that may influence transmission of infection from mother to child. Incomplete knowledge about the natural history of the infection in perinatally infected children probably requires that this figure be viewed as a provisional one (see Chapter 1). There is no evidence that caesarean section reduces the risk of infection from mother to baby[16] and therefore, vaginal delivery should be the aim.

HIV has been isolated from the milk of asymptomatic HIV-positive women[17]. Concern that this may be a route of infection has arisen on the basis of a number of case reports of breastfed babies, whose mothers were infected with HIV after delivery, and who themselves went on to demonstrate evidence of infection[18,19]. These mothers may have been more likely to transmit infection at this time because of the viraemia which occurs at the time of seroconversion. There is no strong evidence to suggest that the babies of women seropositive during pregnancy are exposed to a significantly increased risk as a consequence of breastfeeding[20]. The World Health Organisation supports breastfeeding by the mother as the preferred method where safe and effective alternatives to breast milk do not exist[21]. (See also p. 86 and Chapters 1 and 7.)

How should HIV testing of women be approached?

Ideally, all women booked for antenatal care should receive up-to-date written information about HIV infection, including how it is transmitted and how the risk of infection can be avoided. The HIV test should be explained and mention made of the possible advantages and disadvantages of antenatal HIV testing. The primary objective should be to use antenatal care as an opportunity to raise the health awareness of all women and to offer them a basis for considering whether being tested for HIV has any relevance for their care.

The practice of identifying particular women as suitable targets for information and testing on the basis of perceived risk factors has been demonstrated to be unreliable[22]. In addition, such a strategy may result in failure to provide information and counselling facilities to women not perceived to be at risk, although they might require them[23]. An approach to testing in which the care givers retain the initiative in raising the issue of HIV testing is liable to result in some women being deprived of their right to an informed choice as a consequence of being identified as 'high risk'.

Midwives have an important role to play in creating a context of care which provides women with positive health education about HIV and other sexually transmitted diseases. They need to be prepared in their own education and practice to engage in discussion about HIV with women. This will form the basis for informed decision-making in pregnancy.

Prior to HIV testing taking place, it is essential that the midwife or other care giver is confident that the medical, legal and emotional implications of a positive or negative test result are appreciated by the woman[24]. Every woman who is considering being tested must be provided with thorough pretest counselling in the course of which these issues should be explored[25].

If testing for HIV, it is important to explain in advance how long it will be before results are available (from same day to two weeks) and an appointment should be arranged specifically to report the results.

What use is antenatal testing for HIV?

- For the woman who is worried about having been exposed to HIV, a test which excludes the presence of infection will reduce the anxiety she would otherwise face. It is essential though for her to realise that if exposure to infection was recent, i.e. within the last three months, a second test will be required after an interval of three months to allow for the time required for seroconversion. It is also important for her to understand the circumstances that might expose her to HIV so that she can adopt practices to avoid infection. Explanation of safer sexual activity must be offered and condoms should be supplied. If she is an injecting drug user she should appreciate the danger of sharing 'equipment' and be provided with a source of sterile needles and syringes.
- Advance knowledge of the possibility of HIV infection in the newborn may confer some advantage to a woman by enabling her to learn about and plan for the medical follow-up of her baby.
- Continuing pregnancy with a knowledge of her own potential illness is likely to give considerable extra anxiety to the woman and those close to her. Early access to counselling services and support groups may enable her to begin to come to terms with, and plan for, the uncertainties and difficulties she will face in future.
- A woman with a positive HIV test may want to consider termination of the pregnancy in order to avoid the birth of an infected baby and/or because of concern about her own health in the short or long term.

Termination of pregnancy

For a woman considering termination of pregnancy, the incompleteness of information available about the risks of HIV infection to her and her fetus are clearly unsatisfactory. When counselling the woman, factual information about HIV infection can only be as good as the information available at the time that the counselling takes place. Therefore, it is vital that the person counselling keeps abreast of current research findings.

Some of the important issues worthy of consideration when involved with termination counselling are listed below:

- *Attitudes to pregnancy and to abortion.* These attitudes need to be explored in order to form the basis for a discussion of termination.
- *Gestation of pregnancy.* Of further consequence is the period of gestation when the diagnosis is made. It may be that the pregnancy is too advanced for termination to be considered.
- *Maternal illness.* If a woman has symptomatic HIV infection her life expectancy is shortened and she may wish to consider termination on the grounds of ill health. However, some women may choose to continue the pregnancy despite illness.
- *Desire to have a child.* If an HIV-positive pregnant woman wants to have a child, is asymptomatic and in generally good health, it is probably prudent for her to continue the current pregnancy. Her immunological status and general health may be expected to get worse over time or at best remain stable, and therefore her prospects for a healthy pregnancy are unlikely to improve[26].
- *Social factors.* It should be noted that studies of women with a drug dependency problem found that HIV infection may not be a strong determinant for a woman's decision to terminate a pregnancy[8].

Considerations for the care of women known to be HIV antibody-positive

Breaking bad news

One of the most difficult times for a woman is when she is given a positive HIV result. The period immediately after receiving the result is likely to be a time of shock and intense emotion[27]. She may be unable to think rationally and may have difficulty in taking in information or in making decisions about the pregnancy. It is important to provide the woman with adequate support or a 'lifeline' at this time. Before she leaves clinic she should be given a telephone number where a supportive contact will be available. She may experience despair and might even contemplate suicide and therefore ideally she should not be alone in the period immediately after receiving a positive result. It is a great advantage if she has identified in advance someone to whom she can turn at this time.

The midwife present in the clinic when the results are given will play an important part in organising support for the woman. It is crucial that a further appointment is given within the next few days to give the woman an early opportunity to receive information and discuss her concerns, which may include anxieties about her own health and the baby's risk of infection. Although there are time constraints if termination of pregnancy is under discussion, it is unwise for her to rush into a decision.

The psychosocial impact of learning of HIV infection during pregnancy is unique and overwhelming and it will be important for staff to familiarise themselves with support systems and to develop mechanisms for referral[28]. A trained counsellor should be available to help support the woman during these early stages.

Confidentiality

One of the greatest fears of a woman with HIV infection is a breach of confidentiality. Such a breach can result in disastrous social and psychological consequences for the mother and her infant. In some instances, the woman's partner or family may be unaware of her HIV status and accidental disclosure can put personal, family and social relationships at risk. If confidentiality cannot be ensured, the trust required for a good working relationship with the midwife is jeopardised and there is the danger that the woman will stop attending for care[25]. (See also Chapter 5.)

Policy decisions, which ensure that information about HIV status is restricted to immediate care givers and that the woman herself has control over disclosing the information to others, must be made and enforced.

Many staff, both directly and indirectly involved in care, have access to notes and if a diagnosis of HIV infection is indicated in the notes, either in writing or by some symbol, it may result in a breach of confidentiality. Furthermore, biohazard labelling of blood samples with reference to the name and diagnosis on the request form may result in accidental disclosure which is to be avoided. Using the case number or some code in order to protect identity is a method which is worth exploring.

Aspects of antenatal care

In conjunction with a senior obstetrician, the midwife has a vital role in providing continuity of care for the woman who continues her pregnancy. This will give the woman the advantage of developing a relationship with a small supportive team which can respond to her individual needs and therefore reduce the need for superfluous staff to be involved in her care. During the antenatal period advice should be made available on nutrition, rest and strategies for maintaining optimal health both during pregnancy and after.

Regular medical surveillance for general health and immunological status will usually be undertaken as a routine in pregnancy. Furthermore, there is evidence to suggest an increased risk of cervical intra-epithelial neoplasia in HIV-positive women[29], and it may be necessary to perform a colposcopic examination to exclude this during pregnancy.

Midwives and other carers need to appreciate the possible significance of non-specific signs and symptoms in the woman such as severe weight loss, diarrhoea and oral thrush, and the woman must be encouraged to report any symptoms so that immunological investigation may take place. Furthermore, it is not unusual to see attacks of herpes in the woman which is of additional significance because of the risk of neonatal infection.

It is important before delivery for the woman to meet the paediatrician who will be responsible for surveillance of the baby so that a follow-up programme can be discussed. During this meeting, an honest discussion should take place about the difficulties in making a diagnosis of HIV infection during early life. A particular area of preparation will relate to the prolonged period of uncertainty which will have to be endured regarding the child's HIV status (see Chapters 1 and 2).

Establishing good rapport during the antenatal period between physicians and parents, as well as the creation of an effective and reliable support network, may help to ameliorate some of the pain of the experience. It may also encourage early consultation in the event of ill-health of the baby in the post-natal period.

Preparation for feeding

In the antenatal period, time should also be devoted to a discussion of plans for infant feeding. If a woman who is HIV positive has planned to breastfeed, a full discussion should take place in which she can consider the available evidence for transmission of the virus by this route. Infection acquired after birth through breastmilk has been implicated in several case reports[30,18,31] and by reports of HIV in human milk[32]. In these cases, the mothers seroconverted after delivery and the infants were likely to have been exposed to high levels of circulating virus in the breastmilk in the absence of maternal HIV antibody. The added risk of infection in a child who is breastfed by an infected mother is unclear and difficult to assess, although preliminary results from prospective studies suggest similar rates of vertical transmission regardless of feeding practices[33]. The Department of Health has advocated that 'all mothers known to be HIV infected should be discouraged from breastfeeding'[34] and '. . . they should be advised that it is prudent therefore to avoid breastfeeding'[35]. However, it is essential to consider this advice in the context of the individual woman and her circumstances. Current World Health Organisation advice is that consideration should be given to the social and economic context of the mother and child and whether there are safe and effective alternatives to breastfeeding available[21]. In many parts of Africa, the frequency of AIDS is high in pregnant women but human breastmilk, even from an infected mother, provides the only safe food for infants whilst conferring immunological advantages. To withhold breastmilk from such children would be deliberately to increase their risks of exposure to infective organisms which could accelerate the progression of disease in infants already infected with HIV[36]. Another important but as yet unresearched area is that of the benefits that breastfeeding might confer on the potentially immuno-compromised HIV-infected baby[37]. The debate about breastfeeding is thus very complex and ambiguous and in practice, advice is difficult to give. The decision therefore is best left in the hands of the woman herself and, whatever her decision, she should be supported. Should the woman decide against breastfeeding, it should be appreciated that this may be an additional source of disappointment which she may need the opportunity to express. Other opportunities for close contact with her infant may help to reduce her sense of disappointment[38]. (See also Chapter 7.)

Donation of human milk

The Department of Health[34,35] recommend that potential milk donors in the United Kingdom who intend to donate milk for other women's babies must be tested for HIV antibody monthly, with cryostorage of donated milk for three months until the donor tests negative. Furthermore, the milk should be pasteurised before it can be used.

Preparation for delivery

It is often valuable for the woman to visit the delivery suite and the post-natal wards so that issues of infection control and care can be discussed in advance of delivery.

Care during delivery

During labour, it is desirable for the main care provider to be a midwife who the woman already knows. This reduces the number of people involved in her labour and further protects confidentiality as well as giving additional support within an established relationship.

Universal precautions to prevent exposure of staff to blood, liquor and other blood stained fluid[39] must be applied to the care of all women in labour (see Chapter 12). Because HIV has been cultured from liquor[40], it is desirable to keep the membranes intact for as long as possible in order to minimise the attendant's contact with liquor. Scalp electrodes and fetal blood sampling should be avoided because of the theoretical risk of the infant becoming infected because of exposure to maternal blood through breaches in the fetal skin.

Accidental contamination of the conjunctiva of an attendant does occasionally occur from splashes of liquor at artificial rupture of the membranes and from blood during cord cutting, and therefore British Standard approved safety glasses should be worn by the midwife and other close attendants when these procedures are performed.

Care of the infant at delivery

Provided the baby is well and his or her temperature is above 36.5°C bathing should be carried out as soon as possible after delivery to remove any blood and liquor. Care must be taken to avoid chilling of the baby and the procedure should be swiftly carried out in water of approximately 37.5°C. Immediate drying will avoid loss of heat by evaporation. Well fitting gloves and plastic apron or water-repellent gown should be worn by the person handling the baby until he or she has been bathed.

For a variety of reasons some infants are not fit to be bathed immediately after delivery and thus it is important for staff to wear gloves for handling until he or she is fit to be washed. Should resuscitation of the baby be necessary, mechanically operated suction should be used in preference to mouth-operated equipment.

Post-natal care

The post-natal care provided for the HIV-positive women should not differ markedly from that offered to any other woman. There is no need for her to be cared for in a single room unless she requests it, and separate toilet and bath are not necessary. Adequate facilities must be available for the safe disposal of sanitary towels and she should be aware of the importance of immediate attention to the disinfection and cleaning of blood spills. Arrangements for care should be sensitive to the sense of isolation and loneliness that she is liable to be experiencing.

The adjustment which marks the post-natal period is stressful and daunting for many women. For the woman with HIV the period is likely to be complicated by anxiety and guilt about her baby's health, worry about her own health and uncertainty about the future care and well-being of her baby. Her self-esteem, possibly low already, may be threatened by feelings of inadequacy in learning the new skills of motherhood. It is of great value to her if care can be provided by a midwife known to her, familiar with her circumstances and confident to respond to her questions and doubts. Separation of mother and baby should be avoided whenever possible and care of the baby by the mother encouraged, with advice and support from the midwife. However, if staff are carrying out umbilical cord care, gloves should be worn if there is any bleeding. Gloves need not be used for nappy changing unless blood is present for any reason.

Gloves should be worn for any invasive procedure such as taking capillary samples for blood glucose or Guthrie testing, as these are difficult procedures to perform without contamination of the operator with blood.

The opportunity for discussing feeding plans should have been given in the antenatal period, but if she has not had antenatal care it should occur early post-natally. If a mother decides not to breastfeed because of her HIV infection, it is particularly important for the midwife to encourage her to achieve the close skin-to-skin contact with her baby which she might otherwise miss.

Caregivers should be alert to the woman reporting signs or symptoms suggestive of illness, and the midwife's daily examination should elicit such information. During examination, gloves will only be needed for direct contact with the perineum, lochia or caesarean wound. If exposure to blood is likely an apron or gown should be worn.

The midwife should create ample opportunity for the woman to confide her anxieties and ensure that appropriate support is made available either by the midwife herself, a counsellor, social worker or contact with a self-help group.

Plans for follow-up of both the mother and baby should be reviewed at this time and the role that may be played by the community midwife, health visitor and general practitioner in her on-going support should be discussed. The decision to inform these caregivers of her HIV status should rest with the woman herself, and she should be aware that the information will not automatically be relayed to them. She should be reminded to attend for regular cervical cytology screening and arrangement of an appointment for follow-up can be made before discharge. Discussion of contraception should be initiated before she goes home and a choice should be made of a method additional to the use of the condom. Data are lacking about specific advantages or disadvantages of contraceptive methods in relation to HIV infection but the intrauterine device may not be an ideal choice because of its association with pelvic infection, to which a woman with HIV may be particularly vulnerable.

It is important to emphasise the continued use of the condom as a barrier protection against cross-infection, even if both partners are known to be HIV positive, in order to avoid possible exposure to other sexually transmitted infections.

The woman may not yet have confided her HIV status to her partner and discussion of contraception should afford an opportunity to explore this difficult problem. She should be encouraged to share the information with him, but may require additional supportive guidance from a counsellor to accomplish this.

Special considerations for the drug dependent woman

Women who are narcotic dependent in pregnancy present a special challenge to care givers. The adverse social circumstances and often chaotic lifestyle which accompanies drug use may make monitoring of the pregnancy difficult. Some women are reluctant to disclose their drug using habit for fear of unfavourable repercussions and hostile attitudes not only from midwifery, nursing and medical staff but from other agencies such as social services. The danger exists that such women will consequently be discouraged from attending for care, with serious consequences to themselves and their babies.

It is essential that a harmonious multidisciplinary team work *with* the woman to achieve the main aims of reducing the risks to the woman and her fetus of injecting drug use and ensuring that she receives optimum antenatal support and care.

For most heroin dependent women, oral methadone maintenance is recognised as the treatment of choice, in conjunction with an intensive programme of antenatal care and social support. Even in the best of circumstances, pregnancy is a time of psychological and physiological stress; for women who are drug dependent, the stress will be exacerbated.

For the woman maintained on methadone, it is extremely important to be realistic about what is achievable in terms of methadone reduction in pregnancy. It is critical to give her permission for needed methadone increases before she self-medicates with street drugs. Dosage increases should be offered in a positive and non-judgemental manner. It is far safer for a pregnant woman to take a higher dose of methadone than to be exposed to the abundance of medical and social complications of street drug use[41].

Occasionally, a woman can be cautiously withdrawn from methadone during pregnancy. However, she should be repeatedly reminded that she can stop the withdrawal process if she feels increased anxiety or is tempted to use other drugs. Accomplishing a small reduction in her medication, acknowledged by praise and encouragement can be a major boost to her morale.

It is not possible to predict which infants will have a prolonged withdrawal period. Most babies born to drug dependent women will need a minimum period of two weeks observation for signs of drug withdrawal. Such signs range from irritability, tremor, tachycardia, sweating, fever, excessing yawning and sneezing, to convulsions.

It may be possible and desirable for signs of withdrawal to be observed for in the post-natal ward while the baby is in its mother's care. Should significant signs of opiate withdrawal develop, the baby will need to be transferred to the special care baby unit for appropriate treatment. This pattern of care depends on adequate staffing levels on the post-natal ward. The mother will be extremely sensitive to negative behaviour from staff. Sadly, judgemental behaviour is often displayed by care givers facing the difficulties of caring for a restless, withdrawing baby.

Good communication within the multidisciplinary team is essential when caring for the mother and baby, and in the majority of cases a series of planning meetings will be held when discussions about the future of mother and baby can take place. The early planning meeting shares relevant information and plans a programme including responsibility for prescribing and other matters, such as housing. At the same time, a key worker will be appointed. If there are concerns about the baby's welfare should it be discharged home a case conference will be convened. However, drug misuse alone will not necessarily constitute grounds for these concerns[42].

Summary

Those professionals caring for families with HIV need to ensure that their practice reflects a sound understanding of the complex medical, social, psychological and ethical issues surrounding this infection. Care which is given to women and their families should lay a foundation of information, awareness, trust and support which they feel confident to draw upon in order to meet the challenges of living with HIV infection.

References

1. Department of Health (1991). Press release. *Latest AIDS Figures*. London.
2. Novick, F. L., Berns, D., Stricof, R. *et al.* (1989). HIV seroprevalence in newborns in New York State. *Journal of the American Medical Association*, **261**, 1745–50.
3. Landesman, S. H., Minkoff, H. L., Willoughby, A. (1989). HIV disease in reproductive age women: a problem of the present. *Journal of the American Medical Association*, **261**, 1326–7.
4. Chu, A., Buehler, J. W., Berkelman, R. L. (1990). Impact of the human immunodeficiency virus epidemic on mortality in women of reproductive age, United States. *Journal of the American Medical Association*, **264**, 225–9.
5. Ryder, R. W., Hassig, S. E. (1988). The epidemiology of perinatal transmission of HIV. *AIDS*, **2**, S83–9.
6. Rothman, B. K. (1988). *The Tentative Pregnancy: Prenatal Diagnosis and the Future of Motherhood*. Pandora, London.
7. Johnstone, F., MacCallum, L., Brettle, R. *et al.* (1988). Does infection with HIV affect the outcome of pregnancy? *British Medical Journal*, **496**, 467.
8. Selwyn, P. A., Schoenbaum, E. E., Davenny, K. *et al.* (1989). Prospective study of human immunodeficiency virus infection and pregnancy outcomes in intravenous drug users. *Journal of the American Medical Association*, **261**, 1289–94.
9. Ryder, R. W., Nsa, W., Hassig, S. E. *et al.* (1989). Perinatal transmission of the human immunodeficiency virus Type 1 to infants of seropositive women in Zaire. *New England Journal of Medicine*, **320**, 1638–42.
10. Schoenbaum, E. E., Davenny, K., Selwyn, P. A. (1988). The impact of pregnancy on HIV-related disease. In *AIDS, Obstetrics and Gynaecology*, Hudson, C. N., Sharp. F. (eds). Royal College of Obstetricians and Gynaecologists, London, pp. 65–75.
11. Scott, G., Filchi, M., Klimas, N. *et al.* (1985). Mothers of infants with the Acquired Immune Deficiency Syndrome: the evidence for both symptomatic and asymptomatic carriers. *Journal of the American Medical Association*, **253**, 363–6.
12. Biggar, R. J., Pahwa, S., Minkoff, H. *et al.* (1989). Immunosuppression in pregnant women infected with human immunodeficiency virus. *American Journal of Obstetrics and Gynaecology*, **161**, 1239–44.
13. Jovaisas, E., Koch, M., Schafer, A. *et al.* (1985). LAV/HTLVIII in 20 week fetus. *Lancet*, **ii**, 1129.
14. Peckham, C., Senturia, Y., Ades, A. *et al.* (1988). Mother-to-child transmission of HIV infection. The European Collaborative Study. *Lancet*, **ii**, 1039–42.
15. European Collaborative Study (1991). Children born to women with HIV-I infection: natural history and risk of transmission. *Lancet*, **337**, 253–60.
16. Semprinini, A., Vucetich, A., Pardi, G. (1987). HIV infection and AIDS in newborn babies of mothers positive for HIV antibody. *British Medical Journal*, **294**, 610.
17. Thiry, L., Sprecher-Goldberger, S., Jonckheer, T. *et al.* (1985). Isolation of AIDS virus from cell-free breast milk of three healthy virus carriers. *Lancet*, **ii**, 891–2.
18. Lepage, P., Van De Perre, P., Carael, M. *et al.* (1987). Postnatal transmission of HIV from mother to child. *Lancet*, **ii**, 400.

19. Colebunders, R., Kapita, B., Nekwei, W. *et al.* (1988). Breast feeding and transmission of HIV. *Lancet*, **ii**, 147.
20. Bradbeer, C. (1989). Mothers with HIV: risks to the baby need to be balanced against benefits of breast feeding. *British Medical Journal*, **299**, 806–7.
21. World Health Organisation (1987). *Statement from the Consultation on Breast-feeding/Breastfeeding and Human Immunodeficiency Virus*. Geneva.
22. Krasinski, K., Borkowsky, W., Bebenroth, D. *et al.* (1988). Failure of voluntary testing for human immunodeficiency virus to identify infected parturient women in a high risk population. *New England Journal of Medicine*, **318**, 185.
23. Minkoff, H. L., Holman, S., Belier, E. *et al.* (1988). Routinely offered prenatal HIV testing. *New England Journal of Medicine*, **318**, 1018.
24. United Kingdom Central Council for Nursing, Midwifery and Health Visiting (1987). *AIDS-Testing, Treatment and Care*. London PC/87/02.
25. Brierley, J., Roth, C. (1989). *Midwifery and AIDS*. HMSO, London.
26. Pinching, A. (1987). HIV/AIDS and pregnancy. *Maternal and Child Health*, **5**, 146–50.
27. Miller, D. (1987). Counselling. (ABC of AIDS). *British Medical Journal*, **294**, 167–74.
28. Minkoff, H. L. (1987). Care of pregnant women infected with human immunodeficiency virus. *Journal of the American Medical Association*, **258**, 2714–17.
29. Bradbeer, C. (1987). Is infection with HIV a risk factor for cervical intraepithelial neoplasia? *Lancet*, **ii**, 1277–8.
30. Zeigler, J. B., Cooper, D. A., Johnson, R. O., Gold, J. (1985). Postnatal transmission of AIDS-associated retrovirus from mother to infant. *Lancet*, **i**, 896–8.
31. Weinbreck, P., Loustaud, V., Denis, F. *et al.* (1988). Postnatal transmission of HIV infection. *Lancet*, **i**, 482.
32. Oxtoby, M. J. (1988). Human immunodeficiency virus and other viruses in human milk; placing the issues in broader perspective. *Paediatric Infectious Diseases Journal*, **7**, 825–35.
33. Peckham, C., Newell, M.-L. (1990). HIV-1 infection in mothers and babies. (Editorial). *AIDS Care*, **2(3)**, 205–11.
34. Department of Health and Social Security (1988). PL/CMO (88) 13 and PL/CNO (88) 7. HIV Infection, Breastfeeding and Human Milk Banking. DHSS, London.
35. Department of Health and Social Security (1989). PL/CMO (89) 4 and PL/CNO (89) 3. *HIV Infection, Breastfeeding and Human Milk Banking in the United Kingdom*. DHSS, London.
36. Editorial (1988). HIV infection, breastfeeding and human milk banking. *Lancet*, **ii**, 143.
37. Minchin, M. (1988). *AIDS and Breastmilk: the Impact on Women and Babies*. MIDIRS Information Pack.
38. Brierley, J., Roth, C. (1989). *Midwifery and AIDS – a User's Guide. Nursing and AIDS Series*. Department of Health, London.
39. Morbidity and Mortality Weekly Report (MMWR) (1988). Universal precautions for prevention of transmission of HIV, Hepatitis B and other blood borne pathogens in health care settings. *MMWR*, **ii**, 37.
40. Sprecher, S., Soumenkoff, G., Puissant, F. *et al.* (1986). Vertical transmission of HIV in 15 week fetus. *Lancet*, **ii**, 288–9.
41. Williams, A. (1985). When the client is pregnant: information for counsellors. *Journal of Substance Abuse Treatment*, **2**, 27–34.
42. Kearney, P. (1987). Preparing for the birth. *Drug Link*, **9**.

Further reading

Green, J. (1989). Counselling and pregnancy. In *Counselling in HIV Infection and AIDS*. Green, J., McCreaner, A. (eds). Blackwell, Oxford.

Hudson, C. N., Sharp, F. (eds.) (1988). *AIDS and Obstetrics and Gynaecology*, Royal College of Obstetricians and Gynaecologists, London.

Mok, J. (1988). Infants of women seropositive for HIV. *Midwife, Health Visitor and Community Nurse*, **24(11)**, 458–62.

Peckham, C., Newell, M.-L. (1990). HIV-1 infection in mothers and babies (editorial), *AIDS Care*, **2(3)**, 205–11.

Roth, C., Brierley, J. (1990). HIV infection – a midwifery perspective, in *Intrapartum Care*, Alexander, J., Levy, V., Roch, S. (eds.). Macmillan Education, Basingstoke.

7 The nursing care of children with HIV-related disease

Tony Harrison and Janet Hall

Introduction

To date, there are notably few models of nursing care for children with HIV disease available to paediatric nurses. This chapter presents a model based on personal experience, which is in no way prescriptive, but which may offer nurses an approach which may be adapted for their own use.

Far from being miniature adults, children are unique in their attitudes, emotions, presentations in illness and in their nursing care needs. It is important, therefore, that children are cared for by practitioners who are appropriately trained and qualified. The specific needs and problems of families with HIV infection can then be met with effective care. In the area of nursing of the child with HIV infection and AIDS, it is important that paediatric nurses receive appropriate education concerning the specific problems of the child and family affected by HIV disease.

The UNICEF convention[1] identifies three broad areas which reflect the rights of the child, these are as follows:

- Provision. The right to have access to appropriate care and services.
- Protection. The right to be shielded from harmful acts and practices.
- Participation. The child's right to be heard on decisions affecting his or her life. (This emphasises the child's and parent's right to make informed choices regarding all aspects of their nursing care.)

These rights are mirrored in the UKCC code of conduct[2], which regulates nursing practice and should underpin all nursing care (see Chapter 5).

Children are not the sole recipients of care. Paediatric practice seeks to nurse the child and his or her family and offer the family a partnership in care. The challenge of HIV disease in the family, which may affect many members within that family, may require nurses to adapt their care from child-centred care with family participation to family-centred care, developing models to nurse the sick family together. In the context of this chapter, family will be used to refer to the group of people with which the child identifies and may include foster parents, grandparents, adoptive parents and extended families as well as natural parents.

Nursing, if it is to be effective, requires a structured approach. This structure may take the form of the utilisation of an appropriate model or a particular organisation of nursing, such as primary nursing care. Experience suggests that a framework is vital to the delivery of effective care and will ensure that all the needs of the child and family are identified and met.

In common with all paediatric nursing practice, the right of the child and his or her family to exercise choice in care, based on full knowledge which will allow maximum participation, is of paramount importance. A baseline assessment of the child and family's existing knowledge of and perceptions about HIV disease is therefore an important first step in identifying future learning needs. Issues of confidentiality require the nurse to carefully identify with the family which members are aware of the diagnosis of HIV disease. This is part of the process of recognising existing support systems and resources and ensures the maintenance of confidentiality within the boundaries set by the family.

HIV infection may manifest itself in a variety of ways – from asymptomatic infection to the devastating effects of AIDS. Therefore, nurses need to be flexible in their approach to individualised care.

The asymptomatic child

The child with asymptomatic HIV disease is indistinguishable from any other child, but may be identified in relation to a sick parent, or as a result of investigation relating to some other disorder. These children may be monitored or prophylactically treated in some centres, thus requiring observation and care.

These families should have access to all existing social, educational and health services. Society's attitudes, fostered by media coverage and lack of general information, may affect this right and cause increased stress on the affected family. The nurse involved with such families will need to be aware of available resources and make appropriate referrals, giving support and information thus enabling the families to overcome some of these problems.

Indications that positive health initiatives may assist the individual to maintain a state of well-being rather than progressing to a symptomatic state, may have important implications in child care. Adequate immunisation, health care monitoring, the avoidance of contact with individuals who have infectious diseases and a nutritious balanced diet are all factors which may also contribute to the HIV-positive child remaining well.

The multi-cultured nature of society requires that all nurses adapt their care to meet the cultural requirements of the family. The culture in question may be geographical or social, and the nurse may seek to understand the effects of cultural differences in order to meet the needs of the family.

The way in which a given family or individual became infected may seem of minimal importance in providing nursing care, however nurses need to be aware of possible stereotypical prejudice associated with a particular transmission route.

The effects of the stress of living with a potentially ill child within the family that may have considerable existing problems, including the possibility of illness in the parents and siblings can be immense. The strain on family unit and existing support systems may cause degeneration of the unit unless appropriate support can be found. The role of grandparental involvement in child care has sometimes been an accepted part of paediatric disease, however in families with HIV disease this involvement may not always be appropriate. Some families with HIV may have become discordant and parents may not desire the extended families involvement. A knowledge of family make up and existing potential support systems is therefore vital in planning nursing care (see also Chapter 9).

Care of the neonatal baby born to a mother with HIV infection

The management and care of the infant will depend on any signs or symptoms which may be apparent. If the baby is well at birth there will be no need for any alternative intervention. Paediatric assessment and follow-up is important for all babies at risk of having HIV infection. Symptoms of prematurity, low birthweight, methadone or other drug withdrawal, etc., will need careful observation and treatment. Babies will require investigations, appropriate therapy and nursing care (see also Chapters 3 and 6).

The symptomatic child

The structure chosen to analyse the nursing care of the symptomatic HIV-positive child is adapted from Gordon[3]. This model seeks to assess the needs of the child and family in a holistic and thorough manner by examining the child and family in order to gain an overall picture.

Physical functions

Sleep-rest

The need for the child to have adequate sleep and rest.

Potential problems

The child's inability to sleep or rest due to:

— Presenting symptoms
— Fear and anxiety, precipitated by strange environment, illness and separation from family unit
— Nursing and mecial intervention and procedures.

Objective of care

To ensure adequate rest and sleep, if possible according to the child's normal routine, also allowing for the increased demands for rest caused by illness.

Intervention

  i   Obtain baseline information regarding the child's usual sleep and rest pattern.
 ii   Plan nursing care to maintain this identified pattern.
iii   Ensure that medical and nursing staff co-ordinate procedures so that they do not interfere with the rest/sleep requirements of the child.
 iv   Provide an appropriate environment which facilitates rest.
  v   With the assistance of the family ensure the child has his or her usual rest aids, e.g. teddies, blankets, soothers, etc.
 vi   Observe for symptoms of tiredness such as listlessness, 'heavy eyes', etc., which may indicate insufficient sleep or rest.
vii   Anxiety may precipitate 'bad dreams' in some children. The nurse should be available to offer support to both parents and child or provide comfort if the carer is unavailable.

viii   If possible encourage parents to be resident with the child by providing sleeping facilities nearby.
ix   Ensure that the parents receive adequate rest and sleep by providing facilities and support, e.g. discussing anxieties etc.

Skin integrity

The need to maintain the skin in optimum condition, intact and of usual appearance.

Potential problems

i   Fungal infections (e.g. *Candida albicans*).
ii   Viral infections (e.g. Herpes).
iii   Bacterial infections.
iv   Rash associated with HIV disease, eczematous in appearance but of unknown origin.
v   Purpura.
vi   Pressure problems associated with immobility.
vii   Napkin rash secondary to diarrhoea.

Objective of care

To maintain the child's skin integrity and appearance and to obtain relief of associated symptoms such as pruritis, swelling, soreness, etc.

Intervention

i   Obtain a baseline assessment of the child's skin condition, noting all abnormalities and, if appropriate, measuring them.
ii   Infectious skin conditions will require barrier nursing precautions.
iii   The affected skin surface should be kept clean and dry. It may be beneficial to nurse the affected area exposed.
iv   Appropriate medication should be applied locally and systematically as prescribed.
v   Observe body temperature frequently as this may be elevated in infective skin conditions.
vi   Nurse the child in a cool atmosphere in order to reduce any irritation.
vii   The medical staff should be informed if the child has purpura and nurses should assist with relevant investigations and treatment.
viii   Pressure area care should be given by alternating the immobile child's position. Appropriate nursing aides may be needed.
ix   Nappies should be changed whenever soiled or wet and barrier creams may be applied to the skin to prevent soreness. Existing nappy rash should be treated with appropriate medication and nursed exposed.
x   The nurse should assist the child to maintain his or her usual bathing and general hygiene routines, if appropriate.

Nutrition

The need for the child to receive an adequate diet in order to maintain body function and growth.

Potential problems

  i HIV wasting syndrome/failure to thrive.
 ii Weight loss associated with infection.
iii Anorexia and loss of appetite due to the side effects of drug therapies.
 iv Mechanical feeding difficulties, e.g. oral candidiasis, Herpes, etc.
  v Gastro-enteritis.
 vi Low birthweight babies.

Objective of care

For the child to receive an adequate, balanced diet which meets the needs of the child's developing body and is acceptable in terms of the child's preference and culture.

Intervention

   i Obtain a baseline assessment of the child's nutritional and growth status using centile charts.
  ii If tolerated, provide an appropriate diet in appropriate amounts according to the child's individual likes and cultural requirements.
 iii Provide an environment conducive to relaxed eating.
  iv Involve carers in feeding regimes in order to facilitate maximum dietary intake and assist in the bonding process.
   v Maintain a record of all dietary intake and faecal/vomit output.
  vi Weigh babies and young children regularly using the same weighing device at the same time each day.
 vii For those children with mechanical feeding difficulties, assist the medical staff to treat the underlying cause, while providing a diet which can be managed despite the difficulties.
viii The child with gastro-enteritis may require initial clear fluids followed by rapid return to normal diet when loose stools cease.
  ix Persistent weight loss may necessitate dietary supplements.
   x The family should be referred to an appropriate paediatric dietician.
  xi Enteral or intravenous feeding (including naso-gastric feeding or total parenteral nutrition) may be required. The appropriate care for the route of feeding should be maintained.
 xii Long term monitoring of weight gain and growth in the community will be required for all HIV-infected children.
xiii The HIV-positive baby, or the baby at risk of HIV infection, in common with all other babies would benefit from breastmilk if the baby's gastro-enterological condition permits its use (see Chapter 6). The DOH[4] at present advises mothers who are infected not to breastfeed, but donated breastmilk from very recently HIV-tested donors may be beneficial in exceptional circumstances. Ultimately the decision to breastfeed or not rests with the individual mother who, with access to all available knowledge, may feel that the benefits outweigh the risks. It is important for those giving advice and help in this situation to be aware of the WHO and DOH guidelines, so that the mother can make a well-informed choice where alternatives are available. However, in the developing countries, mother's infected by HIV may not have access to any alternatives. The mother's therapeutic drug regime may also be a contraindication to breastfeeding. Each individual situation will require careful assessment.

xiv   Oral assessment and frequent oral care will be required for the child with oral infections. Referral to a dental hygienist may be required.

Fluid and electrolyte balance

The need for the child to have a sufficient intake to maintain fluid and electrolyte balance.

Potential problems

i   Dehydration secondary to gastroenteritis.
ii   Fluid loss due to perspiration in pyrexial illness.
iii   Oedema secondary to renal involvement.
iv   Inadequate fluid intake due to sore mouth (see above).
v   Electrolyte imbalance secondary to insufficient fluid intake or increased fluid loss.

Objective of care

To maintain an adequate fluid intake and an appropriate electrolyte balance for the child.

Intervention

i   Obtain a base line assessment of normal and recent fluid intake, noting the child's preferred beverages and method of drinking, e.g. bottle, beakers, etc.
ii   Assess the degree of dehydration by observing urinary output, skin turgor, fontanelle pressure, appearance of eyes and condition of the mucous membranes.
iii   Assist medical staff in obtaining blood samples for estimation of electrolyte balance.
iv   If feasible encourage the child to take an adequate amount of oral fluids, noting all intake and urinary output.
v   If the child cannot tolerate oral fluids, an intravenous infusion may be commenced. The nurse should note the type of fluid, rate of infusion and site condition hourly or more frequently to ensure the correct prescription is being infused.
vi   Administer electrolyte substitutes as prescribed.
vii   Assist medical staff in treating any underlying renal disorder.
viii Weigh daily to estimate the degree of fluid loss or gain.
ix   Oral assessment and care will be required for the child with restricted oral intake.

Safety

The need to be safe from potential harm.

Potential problems

i   Immune disfunction causing increased susceptibility to infection.
ii   Potential hazards associated with treatment, including the side effects and contra-indications.

Objective of care

To maintain a safe environment.

Intervention

i Ensure adequate identification of the child.
ii Provide close parental or nurse supervision.
iii Ensure adequate immunisation against common infectious diseases (including influenza).
iv Nurse the child separately from children with other infectious disorders.
v Staff/visitors with infectious disorders should be discouraged from having contact with the child. Negotiations with close relatives about visiting may be important to reduce the risk of infection.
vi Identify all possible side effects of prescribed medical treatment with the assistance of the carers.
vii Assist medical staff in administering prophylactic treatment. These may include i.v. immunoglobulins, nebulised pentamidine, antibiotics, antivirals and antifungals, etc.
viii Monitor the child's vital signs, particularly body temperature, in order to detect early signs of infection.
ix Ensure that staff and visitors are aware of basic infection control procedures and their application to the home environment.

Maintaining body temperature

The need to maintain the child's body temperature within physiological norms.

Potential problems

i Pyrexia (or hypothermia in the neonate) secondary to an infective process.
ii Pyrexia of unknown origin.
iii Febrile convulsions secondary to pyrexia.

Objective of care

To maintain a comfortable, safe body temperature within normal physiological limits.

Intervention

i Obtain baseline recordings of the child's body temperature.
ii Obtain temperature recordings four hourly or as the child physical condition dictates.
iii Ensure carers are aware of how to take accurate temperature readings, that they have the requisite equipment and that they are aware of the significance of variations in temperature.
iv If the child is pyrexial, assist the child/parent to alter the ambient temperature surrounding the child by removal, change or addition of clothing, ventilation and, if required, fan therapy.
v Provide facilities for frequent refreshing washes when the child is pyrexial to promote comfort.
vi Ensure increased fluid intake appropriate to the child's requirements to

compensate for increased insensible loss when pyrexial.

vii Administer anti-pyretic agents as prescribed and indicated. Ensure carers are aware of the safe usage of anti-pyretics. The nurse should be aware that children receiving zidovudine/AZT should not take paracetamol, according to the manufacturer's instructions. Children under twelve and those with haemophilia are not advised to take aspirin, this may cause problems; the advice of a paediatric pharmacist should be sought.

viii Assist medical staff to perform investigations to isolate the cause of fluctuating body temperature.

ix Administer the prescribed treatment for identified underlying causes.

x Observe the child for febrile reactions such as convulsions. Ensure carers are aware of the management of these conditions.

Sensory functions

The need for the child to experience the world through sensory input, in order to develop in understanding and experience of the environment.

Potential problems

i   Cytomegalovirus retinitis (in older children).
ii Visual loss/blindness secondary to toxoplasmosis infection.
iii Otitis media.
iv Bacterial ear infections.
v   Oral candidiasis
vi Parotitis
vii Upper respiratory tract infections.
viii HIV-related peripheral neuropathy.
ix Cerebral lymphoma.
x   HIV neurological disease.
xi Speech loss due to cerebral complications.

Objective of care

To maximise the sensory abilities of the child.

Intervention

i   Obtain baseline data regarding the child's sensory function/difficulties.
ii For children with visual disturbance, refer to an ophthalmologist.
    — Provide a safe environment, which enables the child to function utilising alternative sensory inputs.
    — Utilise tactile and auditory play/stimulation.
    — Assist medical staff to treat underlying cause.
iii For children with auditory disturbances refer to the audiologist and ear, nose and throat consultant.
    — Investigate with the carers, alternative communication methods.
    — Assist medical staff to treat the underlying cause.
iv Assist in treatment of all oral infections, while providing an oral diet which will maximise the use of taste as a stimulus.
v   Refer to appropriate self-help societies for assistance with sensory disabilities.

Elimination of waste

The need to eliminate waste from the child's body.

Potential problems

   i   Diarrhoea secondary to gastro-enteritis.
  ii   Diarrhoea caused by opportunistic infections.
 iii   Urinary disfunction secondary to infection.

Objective of care

To maintain a normal elimination pattern.

Intervention

    i   Obtain a baseline assessment of the child's normal urinary and faecal elimination pattern, including frequency, type and stage of toilet training.
   ii   Regulate the oral intake as appropriately for the gastro-intestinal condition.
  iii   Obtain faeces and urine samples for diagnostic purposes.
  iv   Attempt to maintain usual toileting technique in order not to disrupt parental toilet training.
   v   Assist medical staff to investigate the underlying cause and administer prescribed medication.
  vi   Assist the child/family to maintain skin hygiene particularly in conditions which may threaten skin integrity.
 vii   Provide requisite materials such as nappies etc.
viii   If the fluid or electrolyte balance is impaired by increased elimination the nurse should institute appropriate care (see above).

Breathing

The need to maintain the child's respiratory function.

Potential problems

   i   *Pneumocystis carinii* pneumonia.
  ii   Lymphoid interstitial pneumonitis.
 iii   Other respiratory infections both bacterial and viral.
 iv   Tuberculosis.

Objective of care

To maintain optimum levels of oxygenation and elimination of carbon dioxide with maximum comfort.

Intervention

  i   Obtain baseline observations and details of recent respiratory infections.
 ii   Monitor respiratory pattern (including nasal flaring and chest/neck recession)
      – Colour
      – Respiratory rate

- Respiratory depth
- Respiratory sounds (grunting, stridor, wheezing, etc.).

iii Utilise monitoring equipment, e.g. pulse oximetery, as required.
iv Refer to physiotherapy staff.
v   Obtain sputum or nasopharyngeal aspirate samples to assist with diagnosis.
vi Administer medication as prescribed.
vii Administer and monitor oxygen therapy as indicated and prescribed (it may be necessary to teach carers the practicalities of home oxygen therapy and safety if the child requires this).
viii Provide all care for the child who requires ventilatory support (via endotracheal tube).
ix Encourage carers to assist in all respiratory care.
x   It may be necessary to nurse the child and family while the child undergoes bronchoscopy, induced sputum collection, bronchial lavage and/or lung biopsy.
xi Position child appropriately for maximum respiratory benefit.
xii Prophylactic medication such as nebulised pentamidine may be prescribed. The nurse must be aware of the action and side effects of the medication.

Cardiac function

Maintenance of adequate cardiac function and circulation.

Potential problems

i   HIV-related cardiomyopathy.
ii Cardiac disfunction secondary to electrolyte imbalance.
iii Cardiac arrest secondary to general debilitation or overwhelming sepsis.

Objective of care

To maintain cardiac function and circulation.

Intervention

i   Obtain baseline assessment of the child's cardiac function in terms of pulse and blood pressure.
ii Note pulse rate, depth or irregularities every four hours or as the child's condition dictates. Continuous cardiac monitoring utilising cardiac monitoring or ECG may be required in certain instances.
iii Monitor blood pressure as frequently as the child's condition dictates.
iv Observe the colour of all mucous membranes, nail beds and skin areas to assess the degree of tissue perfusion.
v   Assist medical staff in investigations of cardiac function if required.
vi Administer medication as prescribed.

Neurological function

The need to maintain and develop neurological function.

Potential problems

i   Infection of the central nervous system including:

> - HIV encephalopathy
> - Bacterial or viral meningitis
> - Encephalitis
> - Brain abscess
> - HIV peripheral neuropathy.

ii Developmental delay/regression.
iii Seizure disorders.
iv Primary lymphoma of the brain.
v Cerebral tuberculosis.
vi Cerebral toxoplasmosis.

Objective of care

To maintain the child's neurological function and facilitate development.

Intervention

i Obtain a baseline assessment of neurological function and developmental status.
ii Monitor neurological function in terms of neurological observations, general manner, developmental stage and seizure activity, if appropriate.
iii Observe the child for infective processes, utilising infection control techniques where appropriate.
iv Assist in medical investigations, e.g. lumbar puncture, computerised axial tomography (CAT) or magnetic resonance imaging scans.
v Administer prescribed medication.
vi Refer to and utilise the expertise of physiotherapists, occupational therapist and play therapists.
vii Discuss with the parents the management of seizure disorders and distinct fit activity, in order for them to cope effectively at home with potentially ongoing seizures.
viii Initiate an ongoing monitoring of developmental status, liaising with the primary health care team.
ix Provide appropriate stimulation to encourage growth.
x Investigate the provision of specialist education both within the hospital and in the community.
xi Assist, where appropriate, in psychometric testing (see Chapter 10).

The need to be free from pain

Objective of care

To maintain the child in a pain free state.

McCaffery[5] and Hawley[6] among many researchers, highlight many of the myths surrounding paediatric pain. It is a myth that children do not experience the same amount of pain that adults do and sadly this belief has led to many children receiving inadequate pain relief.

The HIV-positive child who is symptomatic may experience pain from many sources associated with varying symptomatology. The nurse should be aware of the need to recognise signs and symptoms of pain in the child.

Care of the child in pain hinges on correct identification of the cause, source and degree of pain. The nurse should therefore:

i Explore the child's previous experience of pain.

   ii   Recognise, record and report the child's individual reaction to pain.
   iii Seek medical assistance for appropriate treatment.
   iv   Administer pain relief promptly and note its effect.

The use of diversionary play and relaxation techniques together with massage or visualisation should be explored with the family and child and implemented appropriately.

Resuscitation

The subject of resuscitation of children with life threatening disorders is loaded with ethical considerations. It is vital that the nurse, as part of the multidisciplinary team, ascertains the parents' wishes with regard to resuscitation of the severely ill child with HIV disease or indeed intensive support to prevent death. Such decisions on the carers' and parents' part can only be made with full information as to the probable prognosis of any presenting disorder. Support and emotional management of parents' grief are integral parts of nursing care.

It is possible that nurses may find themselves in opposition to medical wishes to maintain life. At this point the nurse must examine exactly what his or her role is in terms of patient advocacy in the light of the UKCC guidelines (see Chapter 5).

Emotional and psychological issues

The need to develop a positive self image.

Potential problems

   i   Alteration in development of the child's self esteem due to altered attitudes of others to the HIV-positive child and the effect of recurrent illness.
   ii Alteration of role within the family unit due to recurrent illness.
   iii Alteration of parents self image and parenting pattern.
   iv Regressive behaviour by the child due to HIV disease and the effects of recurrent illness.
   v   Alteration of the expression of attention, love and affection, perhaps due to family discordance or illness.

Objective of care

To enable the child to develop a positive self concept appropriate to age and development and to enable the family and carers to develop positive caring roles.

The effects of HIV disease and the subsequent attitudes of others on the self concept of the child is a consideration that the nurse should be aware of in planning a nursing care approach. It is vital to assist the family unit to experience personal interaction, and to be devoid of the adverse reactions which have become associated with HIV infection. Nursing care, therefore, must be planned in such a way that families are offered support and positive reinforcement in order to permit positive role development.

Families and children experiencing problems in their feelings of self esteem and identity due to HIV disease, or other peoples reactions to HIV/AIDS, should be offered the services of an experienced child/family psychologist.

Those involved in the care of the child will benefit from the experience of being acknowledged and valued by the nurse and by integration in care planning and delivery. The nurse must examine any innate attitudes which he or she holds that might inhibit this ability to acknowledge carers whose experience of life may differ significantly from that of the nurse.

The display of affection towards the child in appropriate physical contact should be a valued part of image building. The child with HIV disease requires as many cuddles as any other child!

Play is perhaps one of the most significant parts of the child's development and a means by which the child can confront and deal with the realities of life with HIV disease in a non-threatening way. The integral involvement of a play specialist in the care of these children, to assist them in play and educate the carers about the importance of play at home, cannot be over emphasised.

Issues of sexuality

The need for the young person to develop a sexual identity and form relationships with others.

Potential problems

i   Impaired relationship formations due to HIV disease and the potential risk of infection during sexual activity.

ii   Ignorance of HIV status resulting in insufficient precautions with regard to sexual relationships.

iii   Sexual orientation which differs from that understood to be the 'norm' by carers.

Objective of care

To acknowledge the development of meaningful relationships for the young person, which may include safe sexual activity.

Intervention

While it is true that the majority of teenage children with HIV disease at present are those who were infected by infected blood or blood products, this will not always be the case. Sexual experimentation is a recognised part of adolescent development, which has been studied extensively[7]. Nurses and carers, together with parents and young people, need to be aware of the resulting risk of multiple infections if safer sex guidelines are not followed.

Nurses care for children from infancy to adolescence and therefore need to consider the requirements of teenagers regarding appropriate advice and help in this area of human development. An appreciation that parents may feel uncomfortable in discussing this subject with their children will highlight the fact that nurses may be approached by children or their parents for advice on this subject.

Ideally, teenagers who are of an appropriate age and stage of development to begin sexual experimentation need accurate information about 'safer sex' and relationships. There may be guidelines appropriate to their family's moral framework, but should the young adult choose not to adhere to their family's traditional moral and cultural framework, factual advice is of paramount importance. The nurse can help the parents/carers to obtain relevant information that they may require in order to teach their own children, and may support them while they undertake this education. With parental consent the nurse may be able to discuss the importance of safer sex with the young individual. However it is sad to note that there is little appropriate information available for teaching purposes. All information given should be appropriate for the child's emotional and developmental age. [Relevant literature may be available from agencies involved in health education and HIV/AIDS (see Appendix). Ed.]

Nurses may feel that they do not have the appropriate experience or information to deal with this situation. In this case, the appropriate nursing intervention would be to refer the child or family to an appropriate professional, possibly a psychologist or HIV counsellor. In doing so the nurse must appreciate the courage of the child or family in asking for such help. In this way the trust between nurse and family will not be damaged.

In caring for the teenager with an existing relationship, the nurse should facilitate as in every case, an atmosphere in which the relationship can continue and in so doing provide support for the teenager in question.

A difficult area for nurses has been the insistence of parents that their affected teenager children should not be told of their status. In this situation the nurse may feel trapped between the desire to honour the parents rights and meet the needs of the child. Managerial advice and support are essential for the nurse. (See also Chapter 5.)

The nurse may choose to help the parents to come to terms with telling their child or, in extreme circumstances in the light of the UKCC code of conduct, may deal directly with the young person concerned. This may bring them into conflict with the child's family. In this situation the nurse must be clear of the rationale for his or her intervention and ensure that all other avenues of nursing approach have been tried. Nursing management advice is vital in this situation.

Another area which has caused difficulty for both families, carers and nurses is the area of differing sexual orientation. It is accepted that some teenagers go through a period of attachment to individuals of the same sex[8]; it is less appreciated that some teenagers maintain this sexual orientation as their sexual identity[9]. The source of homosexuality and the varying reactions to it are not pertinent to this text. However, the nurse must be aware that tensions in individuals and families may arise from the existence or revelation of homosexual orientation. Nurses also need to be aware of their own feelings towards sexual or homosexual parents, the number of which is often underestimated[10], as a pre-requisite to meeting their individual needs sensitively.

Accurate information about the 'risks' involved in sexual experimentation regardless of orientation would seem vital for all teenagers but, as previously stated, the nurse may well require expert advice on how to handle approaches from children or their carers about sexual orientation or activity. It is essential, however, that a clear non-judgmental approach is shown to all individuals.

Coping and stress tolerance

The need to be assisted in coping with the stress secondary to potential illness and the reaction of others to this disorder.

Potential problems

i   Stress due to living with a long term, life-threatening illness, with potential family conflicts. It is important to remember that more than

one family member may be affected.
ii Stress due to symptomatic disease.
iii Stress due to individuals reactions to HIV disease.
iv Feelings of anger, fear, guilt and disappointment and loss.
v   Possible breakdown of family structure.

Nursing intervention

Nurses are familiar with the concept of 'stress' as applied to the child and family during periods of acute illness, hospitalisation, and day to day living. The nurse must, however, appreciate the increased stress load associated with this particular disease process, due to its family unit nature, the media myths which have surrounded it and the resultant attitude of others to HIV and AIDS. Appropriate and accurate information, which is designed to meet the needs of the family and child with HIV disease, can assist in relieving the stress of living with insufficient and vague information. Nurses should look carefully at providing this information.

A family will cope much more easily if the nurse:

i   Gives adequate time to carers and children.
ii Analyses and evaluates their coping and stress management techniques.
iii Assists the child and family to develop further coping strategies.
iv Offers the assistance of appropriate professionals, for example, psychologists, social workers and counsellors.
v   Avoids giving the family additional stress.

It is perhaps in the area of stress management that the realm of complimentary therapies plays a role, and nurses should seek to offer to the families all resources that may assist them. The effects of reduced stress and positive approaches to health, assisted by complimentary therapies in adult patients, is well documented. It would be unfortunate to deny those potential benefits to the children and families in our care.

Spirituality

The need to utilise personal beliefs to provide support and comfort.

The nurse should endeavour to assist the child and family in obtaining support and comfort from their personal beliefs. This may entail locating the services of a chaplain or assisting the individual or family to practice religious observances appropriate to their beliefs. A prerequisite to this is adequate education on the nurses part concerning the importance of cultural and spiritual beliefs.

The nurses knowledge of the family's social and cultural background plays an important part in planning care for the whole families needs.

The need to have appropriate knowledge to care for the child within the home environment

Objective of care

To produce a discharge plan which provides the family with the requisite knowledge and skills to care for the child in the community. To provide appropriate community support.

It is vital that discharge planning commences on the admission of the family to a hospital unit. The considerations involved are far too extensive to deal with on the day of discharge.

A care plan should identify and meet the carer's and child's learning needs and enable them to move towards self-care within the supportive environment of the hospital in preparation for self-care in the home, and is the cornerstone of discharge planning.   The nurse should explain to the family that there may be possible behaviour reactions to hospitalisation. These may be apparent only after discharge, and the family may need support and reassurance over this period of adjustment.

Preparation of necessary medication and equipment should be made, and the family given clear instructions regarding their use. Follow-up appointments are also an important part of discharge planning.

Liaison with the primary health care team with regard to community support is desirable, but the nurse must always be aware of the need to maintain confidentiality and such referrals as are deemed necessary should be made with the families consent and approval. Consent may be obtained by clearly demonstrating the advantages to the child and family of such community support.

Perhaps the most important part of discharge planing is to provide time for the families to discuss any worries or concerns they may have concerning returning to the home environment and assisting them to identify strategies which will overcome the problems they identify.

It is important for the potentially sick child that carers feel that they can contact the nurse after discharge for further clarification or to discuss worries which may arise only after discharge. An 'open door' policy for these children may assist the family to cope in the knowledge that if any health-related problems arise they can return to the ward.

Planned respite care may be essential for families coping with HIV disease not only for the child but for all family members.

The need to die with dignity, free from pain and supported by those whom we choose

The need to come to terms with the death and loss.

The care of the dying child requires the nurse to support the child and family through the grief of imminent and actual separation. The comfort of the child in an environment of support and love, free from pain or discomfort are facets of care that the nurse can identify as aims to assist the child and family to experience death with dignity.

In planning care for the dying child, the nurse requires knowledge of the grieving processes[11] and the concepts of death held by the child and family in order to provide meaningful intervention.

In this 'family unit' disease, affecting as it may generations of families, the nurse may need to support and care for families with a dying child, or support children who must live through the death of parents or other family members with HIV disease. These may include families who have experienced previous and recent bereavements.

Terminal care is by its nature highly individualised and no template for care can adequately meet the special needs of the family experiencing death. The 'last offices' carried out by the nurse and the care of the body are significantly altered in cases of death from HIV. The Advisory Committee on Dangerous

Pathogens[12] recommend that bodies are sealed in a plastic bag, and relatives should be discouraged from wishing to touch or view the body after death in the interest of infection control. Discreet use of 'biohazard' stickers is also recommended (see also Chapter 12). These precautions may be distressing both to the family and to the nurse. A clear understanding of the reasoning behind the precautions should enable the nurse to give rationales for the precautions to the family. This may help the situation.

The grief of a child experiencing the death of some one he cares about (i.e. parent or sibling) or the family whose child is dying, is inevitably mirrored in the nurse. It is vital therefore that nurses are supported by their team and management in their own grief[13].

Conclusion

In conclusion, this chapter demonstrates the size and complexity of care which may be necessary for the family with HIV. The model used may appear simple, but the disease calls for a holistic and original approach. Therefore it is important that the nurse is offered the same quality of care and support as she or he is giving in this challenging and difficult work.

References

1. UNICEF Convention on *The Rights of The Child*. 1988.
2. UKCC (1984). *Code of Professional Conduct for the Nurse, Midwife and Health Visitor*. (2nd edn). United Kingdom Central Council for Nursing, Midwifery and Health Visiting, London.
3. Gordon, M. (1987). *Nursing Diagnosis. Process and Application*, New York, McGraw-Hill.
4. Department of Health (1989). *HIV Infection, Breastfeeding and Human Milk Banking in the United Kingdom*. PL/CNO(89)3. HMSO, London.
5. McCaffery, M. (1982). Pain Control in Children. In Henning, S. J. (ed). *The Rights of Children*, Charles C. Thomas, Springfield, Il.
6. Hawley, D. (1984). Post operative pain in children. Misconceptions, descriptions and interventions. *Pediatric Nurse*, **10**, 20–3.
7. Vener, A., Stewart, C. (1974). Adolescent sexual behaviour in Middle America revisited 1970–1973. *Journal of Marriage and the Family*, **36**, 728–35.
8. Odiorne, J., Tenerowicz, A. (1980). Adolescent sexuality. In Howe, J. (ed.). *Nursing Care of Adolescents*, New York, McGraw-Hill, pp. 246–80.
9. Burbridge, M., Walters, J. (1981). *Breaking The Silence*. London Joint Council for Gay Teenagers, London.
10. Bozett, F. W. (1987). Children of gay fathers. In Bozett, F. W. (ed.). *Gay and Lesbian Parents*, New York, Praeger.
11. Kubler-Ross, P. (1969). *On Death and Dying*, New York, Macmillan.
12. Advisory Committee on Dangerous Pathogens (1990). HIV. The Causative Agent of AIDS and Related Conditions. (2nd edn). HMSO, London.
13. Kananaugh, R. (1987). Dealing naturally with the dying. *Nursing*, **76**, 23.

8 Part I Caring for children and their families in the community

John Cosgrove

Whilst working as a health visitor with children who are at risk of becoming HIV positive due to their parents' HIV status, the author has become aware that the role of the health care worker in the community is made up of three main areas; liaison, provision of care and education.

In the field of paediatric HIV, the transmission route to the child is important, and consideration for the whole family is necessary. At present, many cases of HIV infection in women stem from injecting drug use either by the woman herself or her sexual partner. Other cases will be found in families from parts of the world where HIV is sexually transmitted and is becoming endemic (see also Chapter 1). Therefore a proportion of the work in this field has to be considered within this context.

Developing mutual trust

The very sensitive nature of the work with those affected by HIV means that a trusting relationship between the family and the health care worker must be developed if an effective service is to be provided. If there has been a family history of injecting drug use there may well have been conflict between the families and health care personnel. Developing a good relationship may be difficult if the family feel that they have been treated unsympathetically in the past. One can understand the suspicion of those who may not always have been made to feel welcome by agencies representing the establishment, when they suddenly find themselves the centre of attention because of a diagnosis of HIV infection.

Suspicion is best met with a consistent, sincere and honest approach. In the first instance it will be important for the health worker to ascertain the family's knowledge of HIV and AIDS. If a diagnosis has been made (and given to the family), it will be necessary to find out how much information has been given. Simple provision of accurate knowledge is essential in order to help the family understand. This two way exchange and communication may provide the family with a sound and trusting basis enabling a good working relationship to develop.

It can be argued that HIV infection itself may be fairly low on the list of concerns and priorities within a family living with injecting drug use. There may be a myriad of issues, for example:

— Financial and debt-related problems
— Housing difficulties

— Problems with relationships
— Unemployment
— Nutritional deprivation
— Custodial issues
— Legal difficulties
— Consequences of discordant family life
— Parenting difficulties.

Before any of these difficulties can be addressed the feelings of the family need to be recognised and acknowledged.

Communication within the community

In order that services in the community are co-ordinated and unnecessary duplication is avoided, it is essential that liaison occurs between the service providers. This should happen at two levels. Firstly, at a specific level – to address the needs of particular individuals and families, and secondly, at a broader and more general level. The purpose of liaison at this wider level enables agencies to identify themselves and their provisions, thus clarifying which services they can realistically offer. When planning community care, it is helpful if some type of forum is created whereby representatives from interested agencies can meet regularly, in order to ensure services are adequate and needs are met. For example, there may be voluntary organisations wishing to provide care, and their strength may lie in offering a flexible service. Unless all agencies are tapped for information, and accurate assessments and co-ordination undertaken, there will be a breakdown in communication and service provision.

Confidentiality within the community

This is a central issue when liaison about a specific family occurs. Full discussion should always take place with the adults concerned to ensure that all possible foreseeable consequences are considered. In some instances parents may not appreciate that hospital and medical records are kept for long periods of time or that health visitor's records are passed on to the school nursing and medical service. They may not be aware of who has access to general practitioner's records or any other recorded data within the statutory sector. Certain areas where possible inadvertent breaches of confidentiality may occur need to be brought to the attention of the parents, because once the information is 'public' knowledge it could well irreversibly affect the individual's or the family's position within the community. Therefore joint consultation together with consideration for the parents wishes is of importance prior to any move towards liaison with any other agency.

Who has a *right* or the *need* to know?

Many agencies in the community may claim thay have a right to know the HIV status of a child, and when the issue is examined closely very few people actually possess this right. (See also Chapters 2, 5 and 9). There are, however, instances when although there may not be the clinical right for an agency to know, it may be advantageous to the child in the long term. Most parents will understand and agree that the provision of a well organised service is in the child's interest. They will easily appreciate the need for liaison with other health care workers who have direct contact with the child, for example the nursing, medical and allied professions. Occasionally parents may have reservations about liaison with others who may have non-clinical contact, for example, nursery staff, play-group workers, those in schools, social work departments or voluntary agencies. These reservations may stem from the parents seeing no advantage in such agencies being aware of the child's HIV status.

Parents of children 'at risk of HIV infection' often seek information about who they themselves should inform. There are no definite answers to be offered to this question as each individual child's case will be different. It is worth spending some time with the parents, if they wish, to explore this issue, as once a disclosure is made it cannot be reversed. All the advantages and disadvantages should be examined and discussed. However, the health care worker has a positive role to play in explaining some of the more obvious needs for liaison with specific agencies, for example, some statutory bodies may have a more sympathetic attitude if they are aware of the full picture. Nurseries and schools may be encouraged to improve basic standards of hygiene and implement Universal Precautions once they have been confronted with the reality that they are going to be caring for someone with HIV infection (see Chapter 12). This may focus attention much more effectively than any number of theoretical lectures, and will also help to dispel unrealistic fears and myths.

When any agencies liaise about specific individuals, children or adults, it is vital that those concerned are consulted and their consent, in writing if necessary, is obtained prior to any contact or referral being made on their behalf. If one agency informs another, or any individual, about a specific person's positive HIV status without their consent it may be considered a breach of confidentiality. One obvious exception to this is when the safety of the child is at risk. In this case the correct statutory procedure should be implemented.

Specific liaison in the community will probably involve the family as a unit, rather than as an individual child. However in many families there may be two generations of people with HIV infection, and in some instances three generations. There are whole and extended families infected with HIV.

Who takes responsibility?

Consideration should also be given as to who the 'key worker' (in the broadest sense) should be. If relationships within the family change, then the health care worker together with professional colleagues may have to decide

— who to regard as family members;
— who should have responsibility of planning care for the children (and family where necessary);
— who else may become part of the team, when consultation and liaison take place.

It is useful to remember that HIV/AIDS is a 'new disease', and there may be a risk of professional over-involvement for many reasons. In some areas there are those who feel overwhelmed by carers and helpers, and in other areas there are very few to whom the family may relate.

The health-worker has a responsibility for checking, as far as possible, the integrity of any agency they intend to liaise with before making a referral. This may be more relevant to voluntary organisations which may not have any regulating authority; but it may also apply to statutory agencies.

Planning care

When planning provision of care in the community for children and families who are affected or at risk of becoming infected by HIV, the type, the delivery and evaluation of care must be carefully considered. Knowledge of the family's cultural background is also important. For example, planning care for a family from an ethnic group may require additional input: the need for translation, dietary considerations and religious assistance. Such a family may be many miles from 'home' and isolation, home-sickness and separation from the extended family may have a profound effect. They may be unaware of the facilities available and need guidance through the social and health care systems of the country. The parent(s) may be attending a clinic of genito-urinary medicine for their treatment of HIV-related problems, and the children may be treated by the local paediatric unit. Effective co-ordination is vital in such circumstances.

It may be necessary to consider the transmission route of HIV in certain families as this may influence the life-style of those affected by HIV:

- Those who have HIV and haemophilia may or may not welcome contact with others in the same situation.
- Those with families abroad may or may not wish to meet with fellow compatriots.
- Families with a history of injecting drug use may or may not wish to meet others in the same position.

The parents of children concerned should always be consulted at all stages, and their views taken into account when planning service delivery.

Clinical nursing in the community

This will probably play a relatively small part in the overall care during the early stages of the disease for the following reasons: firstly, the children who have or are at risk of having HIV are physically well most of the time. Secondly, episodes of acute illness are potentially serious and given the present state of knowledge, it is probably appropriate for the child to be admitted to hospital during periods of acute illness. If, however, parents feel competent to care for a sick child at home, they should be offered every type of support available. This should include care for the child who is terminally ill. Children will benefit from appropriate care in familiar surroundings where the routine and environment is informal and more relaxed, and their individual needs can be met.

Surveillance and monitoring within the community

The child's health will require regular surveillance: this will be a major responsibility for the community health care worker. Where a child is at risk of acquiring HIV infection, there must be regular medical examinations, investigations and developmental monitoring. The intervals for routine checks may depend on:

— the age of the child
— the HIV status, if known
— the need for regular prophylactic therapy
— the stage of the disease
— the involvement in therapeutic trials.

Frequent monitoring may place considerable stress on the family and at times they may not appreciate the value of regular surveillance. There may also be the dread of the discovery of new symptoms, perhaps echoing another family member's previous difficult experience. Venepuncture forms a neces- sary part of the medical monitoring of the child, and some parents may find this distressing, especially if they harbour feelings of guilt about their own previous drug misuse. Some of those who have become ex-drug users appear to develop a very strong aversion to needles and syringes and can become intolerant of such equipment near their children. Extreme tact and discretion is called for on the part of the health care worker, in order to ensure that these children receive regular monitoring. Understanding the basis of fears and concerns of the child and family is important in order to provide meaningful care and support.

Providing a safe environment

When offering to provide regular surveillance of children at risk of having HIV infection, one of the first decisions to be agreed jointly between parents and staff is the selection of venue. As each family has diverse circumstances, a flexible approach is essential. Some will be quite willing to attend an out-patient clinic, many travelling great distances to attend specialist clinics. Others may be reluctant to visit a department where they could be recognised by others. This may be the case for those whose life-styles have been affected by drug misuse in the past.

Families from ethnic communities

Reluctance to attend clinics, where families may meet others known to them, may be shown by families from home and abroad, particularly where HIV/AIDS is prevalent yet a subject of 'taboo'. Families may come from societies where HIV is not recognised with any social or political respect. These families often present in a quiet and passive way and their possible non-compliance with health care may stem from a denial that is inherent due to their cultural beliefs. There are families in this country who know that the care they receive here is very different from that offered to people in their home country, and their dread of being 'discovered' and reported to other compatriots is very real. Some patients may receive treatment for a short time only before returning home, whilst others have lived here with their families for longer. The latter group have chosen to stay here, separated from their extended families, and so may require support and help appropriate to their ethnic, cultural and religious background.

Care for all

Health care staff will need to be aware of their own feelings regarding transmission routes of the virus in order that their care remains unaffected by their prejudices. For example, the quality of care offered to an individual affected by HIV through injection by infected needles, whether in the United Kingdom or elsewhere, should be the same as the care offered to a family where perhaps the child or parent have been exposed to the virus on a single occasion through sexual contact or contaminated blood.

Consideration will be needed for families where the parents may have partners outside the immediate family unit. Confidence and confidentiality will have a vital part to play here, together with a non-judgemental approach.

Community work in different venues

Offering to see the child in his or her own home is an alternative and often more popular choice with parents. This is partly due to the fact that families do not have to travel to appointments and partly because children are less likely to be distressed in their own environment when unpleasant procedures may have to be performed. However, this option may not always be viable – not all members of an extended family living in the same household may be aware of an HIV diagnosis; perhaps the family may be anxious about neighbours observing and identifying HIV/AIDS community health workers. In such circumstances a neutral venue such as the general practitioner's surgery, a health visitor's clinic, a drug group's premises or a trusted friend or relative's home may be utilised.

When visiting families in the community it is important to bear in mind that inadvertent breaches of confidentiality may occur if the worker is known locally as someone whose work is related solely to HIV infection. Therefore when regular and frequent visits have to be made a low profile is essential, and in the clients' best interest.

Attempting to provide such a type of patient-orientated care may lead to suggestions and criticism of providing an extra level of care. The author offers no apology for advocating the most user-friendly service possible, in the belief that it is the most effective way of working with this group of families.

Other considerations for health care workers

Issues for the future of the family

Parents who are HIV positive are often unsure about exploring the options which may be available for child care when they become unwell or die. This is a very sensitive area and one where parents need to decide how, when, or if the subject is to be broached, it may be with a community worker with whom the patient has established a trusting relationship, that the subject will be initially discussed. If this is the case then social services, fostering, and adoption agencies can be introduced by the health care worker.

Legal issues

The parents affected by HIV may require legal help to unravel some of the complications brought about by HIV. There are legal agencies who may offer specific help in areas which may include making a will, help with immigration issues, travel and HIV insurance issues, together with many other complex problems. Health care workers should be aware of appropriate legal assistance available specifically for those with HIV-related problems (see Appendix).

Further issues

Health care workers both in the community and elsewhere may be asked about routes of transmission of HIV. This topic may occasionally be raised by parents of children at risk of HIV infection and the health care worker may have to offer information and unbiased counselling in such circumstances. Many women are unaware of their HIV status before becoming pregnant. Some may have been offered a HIV test in an antenatal clinic and in these circumstances the health visitor may be a trusted person to whom she can turn for help and information.

Communication within the family

All children at risk from HIV infection, and who are regularly monitored for changes in their development, become more aware that the routine checks are something unusual. As they grow older they may begin to question their parents about the reasons for the investigations and observations, and many parents may be unsure as to how to reply to such queries. Some may believe that their child is too young to understand and would become upset or frightened if too much information was given to them. This in fact may lead to no information at all being given to the child which in turn, may increase the trauma of procedures when they happen apparently without reason. It is, of course, for the parent to decide how much, when and what the child is told (see also Chapters 4 and 11).

However, the health care worker's guidance is often sought about how to tell the child what is happening. Parents can be helped with explanations of how a child's cognitive development and comprehension varies with age, and there may be discussion about what level of explanation is appropriate for the individual child. Simple and honest explanations of what is happening to a child may reduce their anxiety level considerably. It may be helpful to ask the child about his or her own perceptions of what is happening in order to provide relevant small amounts of information to satisfy the child's questions without the need to 'paint the whole picture' at any one time.

In some instances where a young child has been told of his or her HIV positive status there have been specific communication problems. A young child may not be aware of the need for discretion and may choose to announce very publicly that he or she has HIV infection or AIDS. The audience, whether on a ward or in other surroundings, may react unpredictably. It is important for the family concerned that they are able to cope with any adverse reactions, should a disclosure be made in such circumstances.

Parents whose children are being monitored may find themselves unable to discuss their situation with other members of the family for several reasons:

- It is too emotionally painful.
- Perceived inability to cope with the reactions of others.
- Insecure knowledge base to offer full explanations.

- Previous family conflict.
- Extended family members may not believe what the parents have to say due to previous family discordance.

For these and other reasons they may choose to ask the health care worker to speak with other members of the family on their behalf, in order to clarify the child's position. If the worker agrees to undertake this role, it is important that the parent gives explicit consent and clarifies exactly what can be said, and to whom, ensuring that confidentiality is not inadvertently breached.

Other needs

These will vary considerably, depending on the family's situation, with regard to the social, economic and physical needs. For example, the health care worker may need to assist with planning domestic help, such as baby-sitting and child-minding, shopping, collecting children from school, home teaching and companionship, etc.

Education in the community

There are two broad aims of HIV/AIDS education. Firstly, to reduce the spread of HIV infection, and secondly, to promote a caring attitude to those who are already known to be infected.

If health education is used as a method of reducing the spread of HIV infection, a high level of public awareness must be maintained. If, however, the health education message is too forceful or inappropriately used some people may become over saturated and ignore the information. Others may take a rebellious stance at what they perceive to be an over zealous attitude by health care professionals. Some may become over anxious at what they see as a worrying situation beyond their control and begin to seek certain individuals or groups associated with HIV and AIDS in order to apportion blame. This, of course, can be counter-productive in promoting a caring approach to those affected. It is, therefore, important that health education messages are carefully formulated to fit the needs of those to be educated.

In the community setting needs for education will vary greatly as there are a broad range of people to whom information about HIV infection needs to be directed. The most obvious groups are:

— Parents of those children at risk of HIV infection.
— The children themselves.
— Their extended families.
— Members of the general public who may or may not perceive themselves to be 'at risk'.
— The wide range of people who may come into contact with those who are known to have HIV infection. These will include nurses, doctors, teachers and social services personnel, etc.

Each group will require a different approach and input, and the opportunities to reach each group will vary considerably. The community health-worker (of whatever discipline) must be prepared to offer an educational input to all the above mentioned groups, together with teaching other interested parties.

It follows that all health care workers should have a basic knowledge of HIV and the course of the disease, together with an awareness of the profound social and emotional implications involved. Parents of children will turn to health care professionals for information, and it is important that this is available at the earliest opportunity.

There are new cases of HIV infection being reported in many areas of the United Kingdom, and it is the duty of responsible carers to be able to provide accurate and honest information.

Community health care workers are occasionally approached by other parents, whose children are not considered to be at risk, to give an update on HIV infection. Such requests are sometimes rooted in anxieties about their children being in some way at risk from another child they suspect of being HIV positive. When consulted in these circumstances, the health care worker is given a perfect opportunity to allow parents to express their fears and deal with them specifically as they are voiced. There is also the potential in these encounters to encourage health promotion, for example, giving information about safer sex for the older siblings or to the parents themselves. There is also an opportunity to challenge the 'it doesn't affect me' mentality which is sometimes encountered. It may also give some parents the opportunity to reconsider any opposition they may have felt about their children receiving education on relationships and safer sex in relation to HIV/AIDS. Each situation will be different and it will be up to the health care worker to recognise the educational potential in each case and act accordingly.

Education of health-care professionals

Educational input for other professionals is of extra value because, as well as becoming more informed, they can be expected to become educators themselves. When working with other professionals, there may sometimes be a temptation to assume that a positive attitude or a high level of technical knowledge is present, but it is worthwhile clarifying the position by giving them the opportunity to discuss their level of knowledge at an early stage in the training programme. It is also important to give those receiving training the space and time to discuss their own feelings. It is generally accepted that HIV/AIDS engenders many strong reactions dealing as it does with subjects of death, dying and sexuality. Exploring attitudes and feelings is essential and therefore should be an integral part of any training session. If professionals of any discipline have not knowingly had any contact with an HIV-positive child or family affected by HIV they may have considerable anxieties because of their feelings of inexperience. Recognition and acceptance of this is important.

This type of education and training may be carried out in small groups, where the discussion is voluntary and the atmosphere is non-threatening. There are a growing number of HIV training personnel attached to each health authority. It is helpful for any trainer to have had practical experience in working alongside people and families affected by HIV and AIDS.

8   Part 2   The school nurse's role with regard to children with HIV infection

Rosie Claxton

Introduction

As there is no standardised format for the role of the school nurse, the work in this field may be dictated by the geographical area and/or the numerical case load involved. The work will include:

- Health surveillance
- Health education
- Immunisation and vaccinations
- Liaison with school-age children
    — their families
    — the education authorities
    — staff in schools
    — all agencies concerned with children, including the school health service.

In all of these areas it may be possible to be involved with the care, directly or otherwise, of families affected by HIV infection. Bearing in mind the complex issues of confidentiality, the transmission and nature of the disease, and society's present attitudes, the school nurse may be in an ideal position to help in preventing the spread of HIV infection.

Health surveillance

All school children receive routine medical and health screening procedures. These provide the opportunity for monitoring the growth and development of children – whether in mainstream education or those attending schools for young people with learning or physical disabilities. Any child who requires further nursing or medical attention will be referred to the appropriate agency. To date, there has been little recorded data about children known to be at risk of HIV, or suffering from HIV infection, who are cared for through the school health service in the United Kingdom. However, there is a distinct possibility that children of school age may present with possible symptoms of HIV disease at school, and will be referred to a paediatrician through the school medical officer.

Children who are infected but remain asymptomatic may develop either physical and/or neurological symptoms that require further investigations, prophylaxis and treatment after they reach school age. In cases where the child is already known to have HIV infection, there may be many health care professionals involved, and the school nurse may not be the most appropriate person to act as key-worker. However, whatever the circumstances, the nurse may be instrumental in preparing and educating those in the school to adapt to and accept any situation involving any children, whether their HIV status is known or unknown. It is important to note that many of the boys with haemophilia and HIV are of school age.

Health education in schools in relation to HIV and AIDS

There is currently much discussion about the spread of the disease in the heterosexual community. It may be argued that statistics[1] indicate that the risk of HIV to this population is relatively low in the UK. However, until further research findings are published, it should be assumed that there is a high risk of infection through sexual transmission. World Health Organisation (WHO) statistics ably demonstrate the geographical spread of the disease and the population affected[2]. WHO also suggest that there is considerable under-reporting of known cases of HIV infection and AIDS.

It is prudent to suggest that the problem for a public health prevention campaign is that if it is successful absolutely nothing happens, and therefore, there can be no room for complacency.

The most effective means of altering the spread of this HIV epidemic is by providing information, dispelling myths, and challenging both attitudes and the risk of unsafe sexual behaviour. It is common to hear the denial of those who think that 'HIV and AIDS won't happen to me'[3].

At the time of writing, all teaching in relation to sex education (which should include the subject of HIV and AIDS) is controlled by law through the Education Authorities, school governing bodies and parents of young people[4,5]. Any person wishing to prevent the spread of HIV in the school-age population may have to present a case to promote recognition of the importance of the subject. In order to enable discussion to take place between young people, it may be advisable to gain the approval and support of the specific authority concerned. It is vital that the young and sexually active population are offered information about HIV and AIDS in order to raise their awareness. This will give them the opportunity to make personal choices and encourage them to take responsibility for their own actions and health. This is necessary for on-going education for future generations of the school population. High profile campaigns have shown a certain success rate, and may have helped to reduce the rate of transmission in the homosexual community, both in the USA and the UK.

It should be emphasised that any prevention work carried out in the early 1990s will not become quantifiable for some years, but the benefits could be immediate, life saving and economically rewarding as well. The argument for such education is strong; the number of those teenagers who could become infected now may have a significant demographical impact on the work force soon after the turn of the century.

The need for education in schools

The need for such education is amply demonstrated in a survey by Canterbury

University[6]. The findings show that young people do require more information and may be summarised as follows:

- Education about HIV disease is needed before pupils begin to be sexually active, i.e. before the fourth year of secondary school.
- Teachers need to ensure that pupils are clear that social contact with infected people does not carry a risk of infection.
- Explicit teaching is needed as to how HIV is transmitted during sexual activity and young people must appreciate the fact that condoms help to make sex safer, but do not entirely remove the risk of infection.
- Pupils must be helped to develop the skills necessary to translate appropriate beliefs and attitudes into responsible action.
- Efforts are needed to counter blaming and unsympathetic attitudes towards people with HIV infection and AIDS.

These findings are from Phase One, and the survey is being continued in a number of schools in south east England.

The statutory sector has not yet fully implemented a standardised and comprehensive teaching package. There are many cultural, religious and ethical dilemmas that could influence this subject. However, many attempts to improve knowledge are being made – through the media, with video films, teaching packs, dramatic and artistic projects and presentations, together with group work and lectures to older teenagers.

A significant impression could be made if the school time-table could accommodate an 'HIV week', with all subjects in the curriculum covering different aspects of the epidemic. Visitors to the school could become involved, and a broad spectrum of people might become interested in such a health education campaign.

It is important to emphasise that all teaching is only effective if the material used is suitable for the age and ability of the children concerned. For example, it is possible to explain the very simple facts of infection and the need for personal hygiene to those at primary school age without causing consternation or alarm, whereas young sexually active people will require further in-depth knowledge in order to make informed choices and decisions[7].

People with learning difficulties

Those working with young people with learning difficulties may have to reinforce simple messages over a long period of time according to the abilities and comprehension of each individual child. This group, already affected by a stigmatised problem, are vulnerable. HIV could pose a great dilemma for them and their carers[8]. There are enormous difficulties in training, and these will be compounded by an 'abstract' approach to the education. Any teaching in this field could be more effective if carried out by a combination of carers and teachers known to the young people, where there is already a sense of trust and understanding[9].

Teaching about HIV and AIDS

The subject of HIV and AIDS cannot be taught in isolation. Programmes and projects may include:

- Communication skills

- Assertiveness training
- Drug misuse
- Personal hygiene
- Education about safer sex and reproduction
- Relationships.

All may incorporate information relating to the spread of HIV and other sexually transmitted diseases.

It can be strongly argued that for all who are concerned with HIV and AIDS, whether in hospitals or the community, honesty, simplicity and a genuine desire to prevent the spread of the disease will provide the foundation of any effective work in this area. It would be easy to assume that this task should be delegated, whether to parents, teachers or other health care workers, but as time and experience have shown, the responsibility for prevention rests with us all – AIDS affects the whole of society.

Working with individuals in the school setting

Whether for immunisation, or for other reasons, most school nurses will have the opportunity to discuss health care in a one-to-one situation. Immunisation by vaccination for those at risk of infection is discussed elsewhere in this text (see Chapter 3). However, it is vital to stress the need for prevention of other infections. The routine vaccinations should be given except where there are contra-indications. This will provide herd immunity (i.e. immunity within the whole population): an important point when considering that infectious diseases such as measles and tuberculosis have serious consequences for a person affected by HIV infection. Chickenpox can also have a serious effect in those with HIV, and it should be well publicised if any of these diseases are known amongst the school population in order to protect those adults and children who may be at risk of HIV and other immuno-suppressive conditions.

In discussing health care issues with individual young people, there may well be the opportunity for the school nurse to ascertain how much knowledge he or she has about HIV prevention. In some circumstances the nurse may be able to alleviate a young person's concerns and anxieties – and give support to them in making conscious and realistic decisions that may affect their future life. It is not unknown for children as young as 12 years of age to undergo psychological treatment because of fear of the risk of HIV and AIDS.

It is also worth noting that in school populations:

- there are many young people who have bisexual parents
- there are those who have haemophilia in the family
- some young people may well be harbouring the heavy responsibility of family secrets
- there will be others who have grown up surrounded by strongly prejudiced attitudes
- there may be a significant number who realise they are not heterosexual[7].

All these children and adolescents could choose to turn to the school nurse in confidence for support and help, in a society which is yet to show general acceptance towards those who, for whatever reason, are at risk of being affected by HIV and AIDS.

Confidentiality for children with HIV in school

Issues of confidentiality are well covered in other parts of this text. It is worth mentioning that in relation to schools the slightly different issues of privacy and secrecy may also be important. There is still a huge social stigma attached to HIV and AIDS which may well discourage parents from disclosing any information to educational staff, regardless of the child's HIV status – specifically with reference to those with haemophilia. It is hoped that the staff concerned will respect the family's right to privacy and confidentiality. The child may not know his or her HIV status, and the consequences of discovering one's own positive status through a 'third party' could have a devastating effect. The child who knows of his or her positive HIV status may deliberately choose not to inform others who are not directly involved in his or her clinical care. This right to confidentiality should also be respected. Those in a professional capacity, of whatever discipline, will realise that the rights of the child and his or her family must be upheld as far as possible[10.] (See also Chapters 2 and 5.)

The young person in school with HIV infection

Depending on whether the child's status is known by anyone at school, and a referral is being made, the school nurse may or may not become involved. It may be inappropriate for the school nurse to offer specific care or support for an individual child for some of the following reasons:

- the parents and child may not wish the school nurse to know of the child's HIV status, in which case he or she would not be able to consider whether it was appropriate to offer care
- there may already be many others involved in the child's care
- the school nurse may not be able to offer an adequate amount of time and commitment to an individual family
- the school nurse may not be employed to look after an 'on-going' caseload of individual children with special needs – he or she may be unavailable for work in the school holidays
- the work can be intensive and support for carers is essential. Support may not be available for the school nurse.

On a more positive note, however, if the school nurse is caring for children known to have HIV in school, there will be many areas in which he or she can help. Practical support may be necessary and a statement of special need may have previously been implemented. The nurse may have already been involved in the provision of resources for children with special needs. There may be physical adaptations necessary, such as ramps for wheelchair access, the need for a quiet area where the child can rest, and arrangements may be necessary for the child to have a special diet, or to visit hospital, or maybe to avoid strenuous exercise, etc. The school nurse is in an ideal position to co-ordinate the requirements that may be necessary for this child.

It should be possible for the child's positive HIV status to remain unknown to others, given careful and complete respect to the wishes for confidentiality. There may be just one or two members of staff aware of the situation, and the school nurse may offer support to these staff members, if appropriate. (See Chapter 4, Part 1.)

Other relevant issues

It is now recognised that there will be asymptomatic young people with HIV growing up through the school system. At the time of writing, many are boys with haemophilia. However, there are other children who have acquired HIV perinatally and through sexual transmission – inevitably these figures will increase.

In the case of teenage girls who are both infected and pregnant, there will be a need for co-ordinated clinical care, help and support from an individual source. The rapport between any young person and the carer is dependent on strict confidentiality. Details of his or her HIV status and condition should only be discussed with others, with the youngster's permission[11]. The normal vulnerability of adolescents can be made intolerable by the sometimes overwhelming difficulties brought about by HIV, and they will need consistent and effective physical and emotional care over long periods of time. It is important that the adolescent with HIV should be included in all discussions, where appropriate. They may well feel isolated, angry and frightened – these feelings may be somewhat alleviated by explanations, reassurance, and the knowledge that there is a carer who is non-judgemental, trustworthy and consistently supportive (see also Chapter 11).

Prevention of HIV infection in school

Infection control guidelines are available from the Departments of Health[12] and Education and Science[13]. They have also been supplied to schools through the local Education Authorities. The content of the following section is by no means comprehensive; the points below echo a few of the concerns voiced by both health-care and school staff. The school nurse may have the opportunity to clarify some of the matters of concern which are raised.

First aid

The guidelines for First Aid in emergencies may be made by the Education Authority in the statutory sector and by the school itself in the independent sector. Most schools have a nominated member of staff who is responsible for the equipment and procedures that may be used in administering First Aid. The guidelines regarding HIV infection state that a universal approach should be used in both cleaning of blood and body fluids, and in the case of any open wounds and skin lesions. If the guidelines are adhered to, it follows that all children (and adults) will be treated in the same way thus leaving no room for suspicion or identification of anyone at risk of having HIV. While the known figures of young people with HIV infection are low, some may argue that there is little need to adopt a 'blanket policy'. However, there is always considerable anxiety if someone considers they may have been at risk of infection, and therefore this should prove that the very necessary education about Universal Precautions is important (see also Chapter 2 and 12).

With regard to bleeding and cross-infection, those with HIV, whether adult or child, pose little threat to others in schools (or play groups). People with haemophilia tend to bleed internally (see Chapter 4.1). The likelihood of their shedding large amounts of blood externally is no greater than for any other child. If bleeding does occur on the body surface, it may be controlled by simple First Aid measures using the same high standards of hygiene with all children. Questions are asked about contact sports and bleeding – the same principles and guidelines as stated by the Departments of Health, and Education and Science should apply. Any skin cuts, abrasions or moist lesions should be covered with an adhesive dressing until there is no risk of cross-infection.

Personal hygiene

The school nurse may help the school staff in reinforcing this subject as part of the teaching of life-skills. There may be an opportunity for the child to learn about prevention of infection through handwashing etc. If there is a health care programme in school, perhaps related to puberty, the school nurse may be involved. It could be appropriate for the nurse to ensure that young people understand that 'blood-brother' practices should be forbidden. The nurse may also be able to ensure that other similar activities, such as ear-piercing, are carried out by authentic practitioners.

Conclusion

The school nurse is ideally placed to enable effective education to take place and to prevent the spread of HIV infection, in an environment where young people are growing up and discovering their roles in society.

The nurse may also be able, at different levels, to help the young person who is living with HIV and/or AIDS. This may be at a time when they would be striving towards independence, self-determination and industry. In reality, they will find they are vulnerable, isolated and possibly affected by progressively declining health and subsequently, a terminal illness.

References

1. Department of Health, Press Release (1991). *Latest AIDS Figures*. London.
2. Sato, P. A., Chin, J., Mann, J. M. (1989). Review of AIDS and HIV infection: global epidemiology and statistics. *AIDS 1989 A Year in Review*, **3(1)**, S301–7.
3. Griffiths, C. (1987). AIDS: The role of education and its implications for young people. In *The Implications of AIDS for Children in Care*. D. Batty (ed.), pp. 56–60. British Agencies of Adoption and Fostering, London.
4. Department of Health, Education and Science (1986). Education Act, 1986. *Health Education*, pp. 5–16, Her Majesty's Inspectorate, DES, London.
5. Department of Health, Education and Science (1981). *The School Curriculum*, HMSO, London.
6. HIV/AIDS Education Research Unit, Christ Church College, Canterbury (1989). *The HIV/AIDS Education and Young People Project*. South East Thames Regional Health Authority.
7. Aggleton, P. *et al.* (1989). *AIDS: Scientific and Social Issues*. Churchill Livingstone, Edinburgh.
8. Davis, S. (1989). Double stigma. *Nursing Times*, **85(45)**, 70–1.
9. Kay, B. (1990). Mental handicap and HIV: the issues. *Nursing Standard*, **4(23)**, 30–4.
10. Claxton, R. (1989). Looking after the children. *Nursing Times*, **85(39)**, 41–3.
11. British Paediatric Association Working Party Report (1989). *HIV Infection in Infancy and Childhood*. BPA, London.
12. Expert Advisory Group on AIDS, Department of Health (1989). *Guidance for Clinical Health Care Workers*. HMSO, London.
13. Department of Education and Science and Welsh Office (1986). *Children at School and Problems Related to AIDS*. HMSO, London.

9 Social care for families affected by HIV infection: including fostering and adoption

Kate Skinner

Who are the families and children who might need help?

To date, a large number of Britain's known HIV-infected children live in Scotland, and the majority of these have been infected perinatally. Most have been born to women who had contracted HIV at a time when they were injecting drugs and sharing injection equipment. Some of the women are the sexual partners of men who had acquired their infection in this way. Although some of the mothers have managed to stop using drugs before or during their pregnancy, some are still using drugs and some of the babies are born with other problems associated with drug use.

Very many, though not all, HIV-affected children have come to the attention of the social work agencies in Scotland. The families are, of course, all different, though there are some features in common which are worth describing.

In the early days of the epidemic, children needed services largely because the family was overwhelmed with a whole range of problems, not all of them related to HIV. In fact it has been remarkable to note that for many parents their HIV infection, and that of their children, has been by no means their most urgent or pressing problem.

Today's problem for these parents is their own disturbed lifestyle, where drug use and drug dependency feature very strongly.

- Many of the parents have poor health, not all of which is drug-related.
- Unstable partnerships between the parents, with frequent separations either as a result of discord or periods in custody.
- Many of the parents are very young and have experienced poor parenting themselves.
- Some have been brought up in public care following abuse or neglect in their family of origin.

These factors contribute to young, inexperienced, immature and unstable adults finding themselves in the role of parents and unable to care for their children or manage their behaviour.

Family breakdown in these circumstances is hardly surprising. When wider difficulties such as unemployment, poor housing, low income, limited family and neighbourhood support are coupled with the fear and stigma of HIV, it is surprising that any families with these enormous burdens manage to cope at all, and yet some do. It is important that professionals keep an open mind when meeting a family with such an intimidating array of problems and do not assume that the parenting is inadequate.

For parents with so many difficulties, HIV will be an enormous worry when they have so few personal resources with which to cope. As the epidemic has progressed and parents have been affected by their HIV disease, their need for help to care for their children has been as a result of their own capabilities being reduced by illness, and is therefore more directly linked to HIV and less to family breakdown, which might have occurred notwithstanding the parent and child's infection.

For children born to HIV-infected women, the pattern of infection in the family may be complex, as will their need for support and services.

- In some families mother and child might be infected but may still appear physically healthy.
- In other families the parents may be well and the child showing signs of disease.
- In yet others the parents may be ill and the child well.
- In families whose infection is further advanced both parents and children might be unwell.

How transmission route affects the family

Transmission routes other than from mother to baby produce different patterns of infection.

- Some children will have contracted HIV as a result of an infected blood transfusion or tissue transplant. In this case they will be the only family member to be infected.
- Where HIV infection has been acquired as a consequence of treatment for an inherited blood disorder such as haemophilia, possibly the child's immediate and/or extended family may also be affected. (See p. 47.)
- The virus can be sexually transmitted. There will be young people who acquire the virus as a result of their own sexual activity, whether they are heterosexual, homosexual, or bisexual.
- As the epidemic develops there will be children who have been infected following sexual abuse. Clearly, work with such children and their family will need to take account of the presence of two profoundly disturbing problems and this will present the worker with an enormous challenge in helping the child and her or his family begin to cope with them.
- Others will have acquired the virus from the sharing of infected injection equipment during illegal drug use.
- A group of children with other particular difficulties will be those born to couples where the father is bisexual.
- Following the political and social changes in Eastern Europe, particularly in Romania, children who have been infected with HIV in a variety of ways, but mainly through the use of unclean injection equipment used for clinical purposes, may come to Britain to live or to be treated.
- There are a number of children already resident in Britain who were born in Africa. Some of these children will be from families where a number of members have been infected in the same way, that is following treatment using inadequately sterilised equipment. Others will have been born to parents who were infected in this way, or through sexual transmission.

All of these will bring with them special difficulties associated with the method of transmission of the virus in addition to the problems of coping with the virus itself and its effects.

Responding to families affected by HIV

Clearly any response to a family facing HIV must take into account the implications of the infection for *all* the family members, including who is infected, who is at risk of infection but not yet diagnosed, and the feelings of all involved about how the infection came to be present in their family. Before a family can move into a phase where they begin to cope with their problems, they need to deal with some of their feelings of shock and anger at the discovery of the infection in their midst, and the very real and urgent need to find someone to blame. This can be a productive area for work with a family but requires great understanding and skill.

Families living with chronic and terminal illness

The impact of a potentially terminal illness on a family is enormous. For some this will mean contemplating the loss of a young child; for the children, it will mean preparing for their own death. In families where more than one member is infected, children may also have to prepare for the loss of one or both parents and one or more siblings. These adults and children will be profoundly affected by the anticipated loss of members of their family and will need considerable help in their grief and bereavement.

Families who have been bereaved talk of how helpful the people were who gave them space and time in which to talk about their loved one, about how much they miss them, and to go over and over some of the feelings of loss and regret. For the surviving siblings of a child who has died there may be strong feelings of relief and jealousy of the brother or sister who took up so much of the parent's time and energy, coupled with a fear that the dead child was loved and they were not. These are perfectly normal feelings and their expression should be encouraged in a safe environment.

The family may turn to helping agencies at any time in their crisis, and their need for services will depend on:

- who is infected
- how ill that person is
- who else in the family requires care, such as other young children
- what strengths the family has
- how well they are managing
- what other forms of help are available.

What services might be needed?

The primary objective for anyone offering help to a family struggling to care for its children must be to search for ways to help the family to cope themselves. Every family has strengths, and building on these strengths should be the first step to take. Support offered by a social worker or other worker from a helping agency may be very welcome to parents needing counselling, advice or just a listening ear to help them adjust to their situation or think through the steps they might want to take. Finances, relationships and the organisation of family life can suffer when people are reeling under a crisis.

Voluntary aid

Practical services, such as those provided by a home help, family aide or a volunteer, might help to ease the burden of running a household. Volunteers are sometimes more acceptable than help from a social work agency and can give a flexible and varied service readily tailored to the family's individual need. It is important to note that volunteers undertaking this kind of work need organisation and back-up if they are to be effective, in order to help them to cope with stressful and difficult work.

Day care

Caring for children can be an exhausting business, and sometimes both parent and child benefit from a short period apart. Play-groups and childminders might be used to give regular breaks during the day to free parents to do other things or simply to rest. If the parent is ill this spell of freedom from pressure and responsibility may be a great relief.

In Scotland, nurseries and day carers (people paid by the local authority to care on a daily basis for children believed to be in need of this service) offer regular contracted periods of care for children. The eligibility for these services tends to be more formally assessed, and therefore takes rather longer to arrange than childminding or attendance at a play-group, but these services may be more appropriate where the help is required over a longer time or needs to be more flexible.

A family affected by HIV may find their need for services changes and increases over time and they may require a more intensive service where more of the care of the children is undertaken by others. Placement in a group-care setting such as a nursery, children's centre or family centre might be useful. Some nurseries are run by the local authority Education Department where the task of the nursery is to help prepare children for full-time education. Social Service or Social Work Departments and some voluntary agencies, such as Barnardo's, run nurseries, children's centres and family centres where the staffing ratio is rather higher and where the objective would be to care for children who may have physical, emotional, learning or family difficulties, while promoting their growth and development through close partnership with the parents. Many such centres organise special activities for the parents to help them to improve their parenting skills. This kind of placement would be appropriate for some children affected by HIV. For some families who wish to continue caring for their children for as long as possible, there may be a place for supported accommodation. This might take the form of support in obtaining a tenancy, where a family is finding it hard to maintain a tenancy on their own for reasons of harrassment, rent arrears or difficulty in managing a household. Having secured the tenancy, the support would take on many of the counselling tasks familiar to other workers in the field of HIV.

Residential family care

Another service still relatively undeveloped is that of residential care for whole families affected by HIV. This would be a good way of keeping together a family who were not managing all the daily tasks of family life, but who could be supported to live as a family in the right circumstances.

Local authority care

Where it is not possible for a parent to care for their children, it may be necessary for the child to be received into the care of the local authority. This may be at the parent's request or it may result from the decision of a Court (or Children's Hearing in Scotland) that the parent is unable to care.

For most children, especially younger children, this would probably lead to a placement with a foster family, while links with the birth family would be maintained and supported, and while efforts were made to enable the child to return home.

If this proved to be impossible, or if it were deemed unlikely that the parent would be able to resume care in a time which was reasonable, a permanent substitute family would be sought. Adoption is a legal process where parental rights are transferred from the birth family to the adopter. The consent of the birth parent is required unless it is dispensed with on grounds prescribed by a Court.

There will be families affected by HIV where a parent is terminally ill and wishes to make provision for his or her children by placing them for adoption. It may be possible for such parents to work alongside an adoption agency in preparing the child not only for the parent's death, but also for the move into a new family. This has been successfully tried in one or two instances, but in others it has been found that the newness of the problem and the general shortage of non-professional carers has meant that social workers and carers alike have been unable to respond as well as they would have wished, and opportunities to ease a dreadful situation for a child have not been maximised.

Day care for children affected by HIV

Like any other carers of children affected by HIV, staff in nurseries, playgroups, children and family centres and children's homes need to be reassured that they are not at risk of catching the infection themselves. Once this assurance has been given, staff have been able to focus on the needs of the individual child and have managed to shake off their preoccupation with the child's positive HIV status.

It is, however, important to note that there seems to be a difference between caring for an asymptomatic child and one who is beginning to show signs of illness. Carers have commented that as the child became unwell they needed help to adjust to the new situation. It has proved useful in such circumstances to help staff recall the work they did in training and preparing to care for a child affected by HIV. An additional problem for some staff and carers has been the deterioration in the health of the parent of the child they were caring for. This has confirmed the reality of the effects of the infection, and the vulnerability of the child to both the likely death of a parent, often the mother, and also underlines the possibility of the child's infection.

Confidentiality

The issue of confidentiality within a group care setting is especially complex. (See also Chapter 5.) Who, if anyone, should be told of the child's virus status? Probably the best guide is to tell as few people as possible, and then only if it is in the child's interest for them to know, and after seeking the consent of the parent. Concern about transmission of the virus in group care must be dealt with as an issue about safe working practices. First aid and health and safety measures need to be well defined and understood, and should be practised rigorously for all incidents regardless of the HIV status of those involved. If body fluid spillages are treated with respect at all times, staff and users of the service will not be at risk. Hence it cannot be argued that professional carers need to know if someone has the HIV in order to protect themselves and others.

An argument which requires careful consideration is that the child is likely to receive a better service if carers are aware of her or his HIV status. One example of this might be where an early warning about the presence of an infection such as measles or chickenpox would give the parent the opportunity to avoid the child's exposure to a potentially dangerous illness.

Early and aggressive treatment of infections may be an important part of the health care of the child and could be managed better if those in daily contact with the child were alerted to the need for this. These points are probably more relevant where the parenting of the child is being shared between the birth parent and the staff in a family or children's centre, rather than in a situation such as a play group. For children in a play group, the responsibility for the parenting and therefore for decision making is with the birth parent, and it would be reasonable to expect the parent to be able to make a judgement about the risk associated with childhood illness.

An important aspect of the work undertaken by staff in nurseries, children's or family centres is their contact with the group of parents. Parents of children using the service do not have the right to know the identity of a child 'at risk of HIV infection'. However, to avoid an explosion of strong feeling if it should be discovered by accident, and as part of a general responsibility to promote good health in the community, staff in all centres for children should ensure that parents have access to basic information about HIV. They should be prepared for the likelihood that at some time there will be a child with the virus using the service. In this way it is possible to help parents to deal with their own worries about the infection, separating this from the knowledge about a particular child. All parents need to be reassured that the staff will be working in such a way that there will be no risk to children in the centre. (See also Chapters 2 and 12.)

The question of who amongst the staff should know of a particular child's HIV status is a difficult one. In some centres it has been agreed that only the officer in charge should be told. It is difficult to see the point of this. If there is no difference in the service the child is to receive, why should any member of staff be told? If it has been agreed that particular arrangements should be made for a child affected by HIV, then the staff who need to know are those in the most direct contact with the child, that is his or her key worker. Staff who have tried to work with this system have commented that an arrangement where only one or two people know is unworkable when there needs to be a sudden change in staffing due to sickness or some emergency within the workplace. Being informed in a rush that one of the children you are about to be responsible for has HIV is not conducive to a calm and intelligent approach. If it is agreed, with the consent of the parent, that in this situation the child's HIV status should be disclosed, then there is an argument for informing all the staff who may be asked to care for the child.

In the majority of cases these general guidelines will be sufficient to ensure that safety and confidentiality are not compromised. However, there are two important circumstances which need special consideration. The first concerns children with diarrhoea. This condition may be present for a number of reasons not associated with HIV. It is a particularly difficult condition to manage in young children and there is often a risk of cross-infection. For this reason, *all* parents should be asked to keep their child at home if they are suffering from diarrhoea.

Another situation requiring extra vigilance is where a child has severe eczema. Anyone, adult or child, in a group setting should take care to ensure that lesions on the skin are always covered with either clothing or a waterproof dressing. This is especially important for those who have weeping eczema. If the skin condition is such that the lesions should not or cannot be covered, then the staff member or child should be required to stay at home until the condition has stabilised.

Foster care for children affected by HIV

In some parts of Britain, local authorities have begun to build up experience of placing children affected by HIV with foster carers and there are now some valuable lessons to be learned. Families who are considering offering themselves to care for such a child have to first be assured that they and their own families are not going to be at risk in any way. Having established this, they will want to know what they may be asked to cope with. Here the agency will need to rely on the good working relationship it has built up with its non-professional carers, so that the foster parents feel confident that they are being given sound and reliable information about HIV from the agency's trainers. They will then be able to trust the agency to tell foster parents when they do not know the answer. There are still many areas where the information on HIV is incomplete and it is counterproductive for anyone at any time to pretend to have knowledge they do not have.

Once families have as much information as they need in order to decide whether this is something they feel they can take on, they and their social worker will need to work out how they plan to approach it. Issues such as confidentiality need to be discussed.

Confidentiality for foster carers

Who should the carers be expected to tell? By and large the answer seems to be 'as few people as possible'. Obviously the family's doctor and health visitor may have to know in order to ensure good health care for the child. Some foster families feel that there are significant friends or extended family members whom they would want to tell. In some circumstances it has proved helpful if these special people were given the same kind of awareness training which the foster family was given, in order to ensure that a consistent message has been received by all concerned.

Very few of the foster families feel able to tell neighbours about the HIV status of their foster child. Mostly they feel that they could not rely on their community being receptive and supportive to the idea of a child with HIV in their midst. Some of the families draw on the negative response they had when explaining or defending unusual or anti-social behaviour of previous foster children to neighbours.

Another tricky decision for all carers of children at risk of HIV, whether birth parents or substitute family carers, centres on how much, if anything, temporary professional or non-professional carers of the children should be told. This is best left to the discretion of the individual family who will have a good idea about the reliability of the baby sitter or childminder in matters of such sensitivity. Asking the question 'why should they need to know?' may help, as will remembering that it is difficult to control information once it has been shared.

Some foster families have the added complication of caring for other foster children as well as a child with HIV. Should the parents of the other foster children be informed of the HIV status of the child with HIV? And what about the social worker of the other child? In general terms, the approach which seems to be the most acceptable is that based on protecting confidentiality, unless there is a good reason for breaking it. If the local authority believes that it is not exposing the foster carers and their family to risk of HIV by placing an infected child with them, then there is similarly no risk to other foster children. In a situation where there is no risk to the children there is no reason for their parents to know. Likewise, there will be no need for the social workers for other children to be told.

The same procedure which operates for nurseries and playgroups applies to schools: if staff follow the well established guidelines for health and safety this will offer sufficient protection, and there will be no need for foster families to feel pressure to disclose the HIV status of infected children. (See Chapter 8, Part 2.)

When discussing disclosure with foster carers, it is clear that it is a subject which is under constant review within each family. Most feel that it would be better if it were possible to be completely open about HIV, but that it is too soon in the history of the epidemic to be doing this just yet. They comment that it has been necessary to invent cover stories in order to deal with certain situations, and that this secrecy is awkward and uncomfortable. This may apply equally to some of the professionals who find the necessary collusion difficult.

When it comes to telling their own children, foster carers have resolved this differently. Some have included their older children in the preparation which they received themselves, explaining that at some point they might be offering to care for a child with HIV. They don't then have to tell their offspring which child is infected, as the issues will have been dealt with in the general situation. Other families have decided to tell their own children from the beginning, and yet others have actually consulted their children about whether or not caring for a child with HIV was a reasonable thing to do. Some families have proceeded on the basis that there is often sensitive information which the foster carers have which is not shared with the family's own children as it is deemed to be personal, and therefore private. All of these are acceptable ways of dealing with a sensitive and complex area and while one way will suit one family, it may not suit another. It is helpful therefore if the professionals make themselves available to help foster carers work out for their own family which is the best approach for them.

Other issues of foster care

In describing how they experienced caring for a child with HIV, it soon becomes apparent that foster carers very quickly overcome their preoccupation with worries about the virus itself. They focus on the child's needs, although the knowledge about the child's HIV status is always there but not dwelt on. The frequent medical tests to monitor the health and development of children with HIV are constant reminders of the uncertain future for these children and for the carers, and tends to lead to a swinging between optimism and sadness depending on what the latest piece of news has been. In the early days of placing children affected by HIV with foster families, the information from the USA (at that point the only experience there was to call on) suggested that the outlook for children born to HIV-infected women was very poor indeed. Foster families saw themselves as preparing to care for a child who would amost certainly become very ill while still a small baby. Much of the work with these foster carers has been around the need to ready themselves for the loss of the child, probably after a period of distressing and painful illness. As time has passed, many of the children have remained well and families have needed to review their coping mechanisms and adjust to a new situation where optimism seems more appropriate. This needs to be tempered with some caution in the light of recent research findings, particularly from the USA, where many children are developing signs of HIV disease following some years during which they appeared to be uninfected. Without exception the foster carers all talk about the problems of living with uncertainty. This applies equally to birth parents who are caring for their own children in their own homes. Many foster families live with uncertainty in the form of an insecure or unresolved legal situation surrounding the children who are placed with them. Foster carers are well used to dealing with uncertainty about the health of children placed with them, but these concerns would rarely be of the magnitude of the uncertainty surrounding HIV. This particular aspect of the placements did appear to influence the strength of commitment to the child and led most of the foster carers to consider offering a permanent placement, even though the original basis for the placement had been temporary. Some families inappropriately offered a permanent placement and considerable skill was required to help the family look again at both its motivation and its capacity to cope in the long term.

Talking with foster carers about the support which has been helpful to them while looking after a child affected by HIV, inevitably focussed on access to medical advice. This was important for a number of reasons. Firstly to establish the HIV status of the child. The difficulty of obtaining a clear indication as to whether or not the child has been infected *in utero* means that children are regularly and frequently tested. All families, including the child's own family, are understandably preoccupied with the outcome of the tests and need to be assured that they will be informed quickly about the results. They need to feel that their clinician is reliable and will explain the implications to them in language which they can understand. (See also Chapters 2 and 3.)

The variable presentation of HIV disease and the unpredictable onset of AIDS leaves all carers of children affected by HIV anxious about the children's health and unclear about the significance they should attribute to any signs of illness. Minor ailments assume unreasonable proportions, and although this is easy enough to recognise in retrospect, keeping them in perspective at the time is much harder. Several families talk of the first runny nose which had led to the question 'Is this it?'

The short shelf life of information about HIV, due to the rapid increase in understanding, experience and research, creates a kind of insecurity which is best managed by ready and easy access to an authoritative source. This is usually, but not invariably, a clinician. Some families are clear that they use and value more than one such source including their social worker, the local authority's HIV Co-ordinator, and a drugs worker.

In a situation where some might say that a child's future had been jeopardised by the actions of a parent, it is not hard to see how someone caring for a child might blame the birth parent for the child's HIV infection. Surprisingly, the majority of foster carers do not express anger against the parents but were in fact sympathetic towards them. For some children placed in foster care there is little or no contact with birth parents. Other carers manage to sustain lengthy periods of visits to the parents in prison, never an easy thing to do under any circumstances. One remarkable family has succeeded in keeping the child in touch with both parents who have been in different prisons many miles apart.

Some foster carers are able to build up a constructive relationship with members of the child's extended family, usually grandparents. It is worthwhile pointing out here that the presence of HIV in a family may, with parental consent, lead to a new role for grandparents. People in their middle years who are the parents of a young adult with HIV talk about the pain of preparing to bury their offspring, and if he or she also has children with HIV, burying their grandchildren too. Sometimes the distress of seeing these young adults terminally ill has led the grandparents to offer to assume the care of their grandchildren. In some cases this will be an excellent arrangement, but in others it will not. Some birth parents may not wish for this contact as a result of unresolved difficulties arising out of their own childhood. For some, it may present an opportunity to right some of the wrongs of the upbringing the grandparents gave to the adult who, if a drug user, has failed to live up to their expectations. This can be fraught with problems and careful counselling is required to secure proper care for the child while leaving the grandparents with as much self-respect as possible.

Foster carers have worried long and hard about how to explain to a young child that she or he has or might have HIV. This is an aspect which needs to be covered very fully in the preparation for becoming a foster carer of a child affected by HIV, but even so the family will need to go over it a number of times subsequently. Ultimately, each family will find its own way of tackling this problem, and there is probably no right way of carrying this out. However, there are a number of wrong ways of explaining the situation, and it is in helping a family to steer round these problems that a social worker or other skilled counsellor can be most useful. As with the disclosure of other important and sensitive information to children, giving small pieces of the story at a time makes it easier for a child to grasp, and also allows carers to offer reassurance about the child being loved, needed and in no way to blame for the situation. Many years of careful study have shown that it is better for a child to grow up knowing about her or his background than to discover this in later years. This does, of course, raise the issue of self-disclosure, and carers will need to discuss this fully with the child in order to avoid a subsequent crisis.

Foster carers who offer to care for a child on a temporary basis do so best when they have a clear appreciation of what the next step for the child is likely to be. A major anxiety for foster parents preparing a child affected by HIV for adoption has been whether or not it would be possible to find adoptive parents for the children. So far it has proved to be possible, but the numbers of children are still quite small. Even so, for some children the process has taken some time, longer than for children of the same age who did not have a risk of HIV. For very young children this delay can be worrying, and it is often the foster carers who feel it most acutely.

Despite all these complications and difficulties, most of the foster families report the experience of caring for a child affected by HIV as a positive one, and most say they would do it again. Indeed some families have cared for more than one child. All have valued the extra support they were offered by their social work agencies, and have commented that they wished the same level of support could be available to them for all placements – an interesting point that workers who link with foster carers might not be surprised to note! For some foster families the high profile they receive within their local authority has an important spin-off. They comment that they felt valued and appreciated in a way which had not been their experience previously as foster carers. The newness of the task and the kudos of pioneering a new project reaffirmed their skills and boosted their self-esteem. Again there is a message in this for those who run a fostering service.

Recruitment and preparation of foster carers and adopters

It is important to remember that foster carers and prospective adopters have a choice about whether or not to be foster carers. This means that they need to be given enough information about the task they are being asked to do, together with the uncertainties, so that they can decide for themselves if this is something that is right for their family. So far, as with placements for most 'hard to place' children, many of the families who put themselves forward are child-centred families who have already had some of their parenting needs met, probably by looking after their own children. This may be associated with the fact that most people who want to parent anticipate caring for a child from a very early stage right through to adulthood. It cannot be assumed that a child affected by HIV will reach adulthood, so people who have not had their own children may not wish to take the chance that their parenting may be cut short. This is not universally the case, but does seem to have been a factor. Another similarity between carers of children affected by HIV and those for children with other serious problems is that many of the families have had to face and cope with a variety of other difficulties in their lives. It may be that the process of resolving their own problems strengthens a family in such a way that they feel able to tackle other difficult situations.

The adoption of children affected by HIV

So far, a small number of children affected by HIV have been placed for adoption. Some of these children were placed at a stage where their HIV status was not clear, so they were described as 'at risk of HIV'. Others have been placed with their prospective adopters at a point when it was clear that they had HIV. A very small number of children were already showing signs of HIV disease when they were placed and are now very ill. The adopters for these children came in a variety of ways to the agency which arranged the placements. Some prospective adopters were specifically recruited for the placement of an HIV-infected child. Others were from a group of families who intitially applied to adopt an 'ordinary' child, and then became interested in a child affected by HIV. Another small group of adoption placements have grown from what were initially intended to be foster placements. In these situations, as the child's need changed from a temporary short term place-ment to a permanent substitute family, the foster family's commitment to the child led them to offer to care permanently for him or her. In some circumstances such an offer might be inappropriate because the placing agency may not consider this to be in the child's best interest. Understandably, this may lead to tension within the placement and between the agency and the foster carers. While there has so far been insufficient experience of these placements on which to base recommendations, the possibility that this may occur might be borne in mind by placing agencies and workers. In general, the feelings reported by adopters of children affected by HIV are remarkably similar to those of foster carers: they do not focus on HIV every minute of every day but it is constantly in the background. They yearn for reassurance from their clinician, but find the appointments and the attendant medical examinations intrusive and distressing. Their views about disclosure about HIV are virtually identical to those of foster carers; they rarely tell neighbours and friends but usually tell members of their extended family.

Adopters of children affected by HIV are protective towards their children, but are conscious of the dangers of overprotection. They are all keen to afford a normal upbringing but each family has their individual interpretation of this. None regret the steps they have taken so far.

Residential care for children affected by HIV

Residential care in either a children's home or hostel may be used for a temporary or long term placement for a child or young person for whom a family placement is either unsuitable or unlikely to be found. This usually applies to older children who have an important connection to their own family or whose problems are such that they are unlikely to settle in a substitute family. From the point of view of the risk of cross-infection of HIV among people living in group care settings, there is no reason why a person with HIV should not live in residential care.

There may be a number of problems associated with the difficulty of maintaining confidentiality when people live so closely together. There can be *no* grounds for informing young people about the HIV status of their peers and it should be made clear to them that they will not be told. It will be of paramount importance that time is spent with a young person with HIV to help him or her consider who they would like to tell, and the implications of this should be explored.

An anxiety for staff working with teenagers in group care concerns sexual activity. If young people are sexually active they need to be taught how to behave in order to keep themselves safe from the risk of HIV infection. The same message, which will protect them outside the children's home, will keep them safe if they have sex with another resident. It is important that children appreciate the seriousness of HIV and their responsibility to themselves and to their peers.

A further issue for those working with teenagers is the tricky one of ensuring that as well as knowing what precautions to take, they also have the means to protect themselves. This is a particularly difficult area, as staff will not want to be seen to condone sexual activity, especially if the young people are under the legal age of consent. Children and young people with learning difficulties will need education and preparation appropriate to their ability to understand and implement measures which will keep themselves and others safe. Social work agencies have never found this subject easy to deal with, but the emergence of HIV makes it imperative that it is discussed within the children's home and a way forward found. Managers will therefore need to discuss and decide how they wish to deal with this very sensitive topic, and will need to make clear their support for staff and their actions.

Testing of children thought to be at risk of HIV

Before deciding whether or not there is need to test a child, it is helpful to consider first of all if there is a strong indication that a child might be infected. (See also Chapter 2.) Suspicion that a mother might have injected an illegal substance would not on its own constitute a strong indication that she may have been at risk of HIV infection. Discussing the need for a child to come into care with the mother might elucidate further information, such as whether she had ever to her knowledge engaged in a risk activity, or if she had ever had reason to think she might be infected.

If there is a risk that the child might be infected, what would be the reason for wanting to know the child's status? Foster carers and prospective adopters have a right to expect full information about the health of the children they care for, and there are good reasons concerned with the health care of the child which would merit their being informed about the presence of HIV infection, if this was known. For many services, such as admission to a nursery, children's home or hostel, it is not necessary for the staff to know of a child's HIV status. Concern about the extremely low risk of transmission within such a setting must be dealt with by good, universal measures of hygiene rather than by the identification of those who are infected or who are at risk of infection.

If a child receiving a service became ill *and there was no other explanation*, consideration might be given to seeking the consent of the parent to test the child, as it would clearly be in the child's interest that a diagnosis be made as swiftly as possible in order to ensure appropriate clinical care.

In summary, the only circumstances where testing of children should be considered is where it would be in the interest of the child for his or her HIV status to be known. Desire on the part of caring staff to know is not sufficient reason to seek to test a child.

Teenagers in care may be exposed to risk of HIV infection as a result of risk activities such as unprotected sex or use of shared injection equipment. If they are concerned about their HIV status they should be given access to high quality counselling about the implications of taking the test. If after receiving counselling they would like to be tested, this is their right to choose as with all young people whether in care or not, and it should be made possible for them to have the test having made their own informed decision.

Some prospective adopters have raised their concern about the possibility that a child placed with them for adoption may be infected. Clearly there can be no guarantees that this is not the case, but it would be undesirable to test every child or every mother placing her child for adoption in order to satisfy this concern. A selective approach would seem to be the best one in this circumstance. All women who wish to place their babies for adoption should give a detailed history of themselves to the adoption agency before the baby is born. If this history revealed that there was a likelihood of the mother having been exposed to HIV, it would be worthwhile to explore this with her in order to obtain a clearer picture. If it was felt that there was a reasonable chance that she had been exposed, then this should be discussed with her before arranging for her to receive pre-test counselling. If she was thought to be at risk of HIV but refused to be tested, or she was found to be HIV positive, the child would need to be placed as 'at risk of HIV infection'. It would not be possible to test the child without her consent until the adoption order had been made, when the adopters would be the legal parents of the child and could therefore give their consent.

It should be said that so far, the overwhelming majority of parents have been helpful when there has been a query over the HIV status of their children. Even the parents who are normally regarded as less co-operative have responded well to such approaches, as it is clear that they wish to do the best they can for their children.

Preparation, training and support for staff and carers

Managers have a responsibility to their staff and carers on three levels. As a good employer of staff and carers, the helping agency should ensure that they are given sufficient information about HIV so that they know how to protect themselves and their family from the infection. Secondly, staff and carers need to have enough knowledge to ensure that they work in such a way that they do not permit transmission in the workplace or in their home. Finally, they need to know the implications of HIV so that they are able to offer a sensitive and comprehensive service to someone who has the infection.

This kind of training programme should be available throughout the whole of the helping agency and needs to be systematically undertaken and should make provision for updating, not simply because our understanding of HIV is growing, but because people forget information they are not called upon to use regularly.

The content of training will need to be tailored to the tasks people are required to carry out, but should include information for everyone about the infection, how it is transmitted, and basic health and safety measures which should be carried out at all times. It is important that time is given for the expression of fears about the disease, as people do not hear what is said if they are preoccupied with their own anxieties.

Working with sick and dying people is very stressful and demanding, and while these stresses cannot be entirely avoided, it is important that these are recognised, and that help and support in dealing with them is given.

When trying to anticipate this kind of situation, it can be helpful to ask people to imagine the most difficult circumstances they may be asked to cope with: if a personal colleague or client/patient was dying, and what might be the most rewarding or satisfying area of this work. This encourages participants to see what would be the worst and the best side of caring, and they can begin to imagine the range of possibilities in between.

Once people have started to think about these matters, it becomes easier to work out ways of dealing with them. Group discussions are particularly useful as a way of generating ideas about such strategies, and once people are into the swing of seeing themselves as having a constructive role, new areas for further learning such as relaxation methods, taking exercise, and setting limits for themselves and others can be explored.

There is a danger that staff may become over involved in the situations of their clients/patients so it is important that boundaries and limits are set. This protects both the professional carers and the client/patient. It is important to recognise that they are best negotiated with the client/patient to avoid misconceptions about the professional carer's role. This will also make it easier for the boundaries to be kept.

In learning to work alongside someone who has HIV, it is essential to be aware of the feelings of those close to that person. The stigma and unpleasantness of the infection can arouse strong emotions, and it may be very hard for family members to continue to support someone with HIV without a great deal of support themselves.

Support groups for those caring for people with HIV have been found to be successful in providing a forum for professional and non-professional carers to share their feelings, to identify with others and to receive support in appropriate group settings (see Appendix). Good professional support to such groups is important, and they should be facilitated by someone experienced in group work, who is knowledgeable about HIV and who has access to informed back-up themselves. Most people involved with HIV are well informed about the infection themselves, but are also keen to improve their knowledge and understanding. Contact with an approachable and experienced person who may be linked to the support group is invaluable.

Principles for service provision

Families approaching an agency for help need to be assured that the staff who are in touch with them have the child's interests as their first priority. Decisions about the kind of service they need and about how that will be provided will be made on that basis, and not on the basis of what may suit the agency best. This is an easy principle to state, and largely we believe that we operate with this in mind all the time. However, there have been many examples in health care and social work settings where the presence of HIV infection has led to delays in treatment or provision of a service in order to take account of the fears about cross-infection where there was no risk to the safety of others.

The range of services for families where there is an HIV-infected person should be the same as that available to any family. There is no need to restrict choice because of HIV. The implication of this issue for service providers is of course that all staff and carers, whatever their work setting, should be prepared for the day when they are either asked to include someone who has HIV, or when they discover that someone to whom they have been offering a service has HIV.

Services need to be visible and accessible and unfortunately these are not qualities usually attributable to local authorities, as the limit on resources inevitably leads to caution about publicly promoting services.

Flexibility is an important issue where need for services is generated by an infection such as HIV with its long incubation period, variable onset and presentation of illness, and where periods of reasonable health occur between episodes of acute illness. Services need to be designed so that users may move with ease between different provisions as their need dictates.

For families whose time together may be shorter than they had imagined as a result of HIV, strenuous efforts should be made to improve the quality of their time together and to involve the parents in as many of the decisions about their children as possible. Account must be taken of the parents' wishes for their children, and their help enlisted in easing the children's adjustment to their own infection and to that of the parents.

Much of the attention given to HIV has placed it in a medical framework, but HIV is not merely a health issue. It has important implications for family and social life. In parts of the country where the epidemic is already well established, professionals from all the helping and caring agencies across a wide field have found new ways of working together in facing up to the new problems of this disease. This could not have been achieved without a great deal of hard work and energy being devoted simply to working together, and this *must* continue.

Collaboration between agencies at political and managerial level, together with those at every other level, is the only way forward. This can only be carried out if old rivalries are set aside and claims to power, territory and professional boundaries are abandoned in the interest of finding the common ground – the provision of the best possible service for children and families affected by HIV.

Further reading

Batty, D. (ed.) (1987). *Implications of HIV and AIDS for Children in Care*, BAAF, London.

Hollins, S., Sireling, L. (1990). *When Mum Died, When Dad Died*, St George's Hospital and Silent Books, Cambridge.

Judd, D. (1989). *Give Sorrow Words, Working with a Dying Child*, Free Association Books, London.

Richardson, D. (1987). *Women and AIDS*, Pandora, London.

Rieder, I., Ruppelt, P. (ed.) (1989). *Matters of Life and Death*, Virago, London.

Robertson, J. (1989). *Separation and the Very Young*, Free Association Books, London.

The Children Act (1989). HMSO, London.

Yelding, D. (ed.) (1990). *Caring for Someone with AIDS*, Hodder and Stoughton, London.

10 Neuropsychological assessment of children with HIV infection

Rebekah Lwin

The neurological concomitants of HIV infection and AIDS have been extensively reported in the literature[1,2,3,4,5,6]. However, they are frequently described as clinical observations of deteriorating function, the progression of neurological signs and symptoms during the course of infection and illness and, more specifically, during the course of treatment, and their precise effect on children has not been well documented.

Clinically, infection of the central nervous system by HIV may be characterised by microcephaly, seizures, pyramidal tract signs, extra-pyramidal and cerebellar signs. The functional effect on the child may lead to delays in developmental milestones and a general deterioration in aspects of cognitive and motor abilities. (See also Chapter 3.)

The precise degree of neurological impairment will vary from child to child and likewise the course of deterioration may follow a static, slow, rapid or intermittent progression. It is probable that there are a number of factors which are significant here, though exactly what their individual and collective contributions are, is as yet unclear.

Factors which may determine neurological impairment

The age of the child at the onset of HIV infection

Where HIV infects the central nervous system (CNS), the effect on the child will be different according to the stage of development of the CNS at the time of its infection. Whilst the CNS is still developing in younger children, the most common neurological signs are delay or loss of motor milestones and more rarely language delay and impairment. In older children impairments of perceptual-motor function, attention and memory are more commonly reported.

Route of transmission

Children born to seropositive mothers, by definition, stand a greater likelihood of early CNS invasion than those infected later in life by other routes, such as contaminated blood products. However, it is important to remember that not all vertically infected children will show neurological signs at an early stage. There appears to be a bimodal distribution of age at the onset of symptoms, including neurological symptoms, with a number of infected children remaining symptom free for many years while others can become symptomatic within their first 12 months. (See also Chapter 1.)

Non-HIV factors which may affect neurological development

There are a number of other factors such as drug use in seropositive pregnant women which may also have a direct effect on the central nervous system of the developing fetus and which may, in addition, render a child more susceptible to further damage by HIV.

Understanding more fully this process of neurological impairment in children with HIV infection and which factors may be significant requires systematic and regularly repeated assessment. Symptomatic and asymptomatic infected children should be assessed in a number of neurological, psychological and developmental areas of functioning from the earliest possible time of suspected diagnosis (at birth for those born to seropositive mothers) and throughout the duration of their infection.

It is too early to know exactly what areas should be explored, but from clinical observations the neuropsychological factors that might require assessment and prospective investigation include the following:

- general physical development
- intellectual development
- language
- attention
- memory
- fine and gross motor function
- aspects of behaviour.

The tests used must have good discriminating power and should also be comparable across a wide age range. This latter point poses a problem as many commonly used standardised tests have relatively small age ranges over which norms are available. Difficulties therefore arise when assessing children over time as the age appropriate test will change as the child grows older and it may not be meaningful to relate results from different tests. It is also important to be aware that many of those children currently affected by HIV infection come from differing cultural and ethnic backgrounds and care must therefore be taken to select tests that do not discriminate against such groups.

Another practical point to take into consideration when assessing children is that of the practice effects gained when the same test is administered repeatedly over a period of time. A balance needs to be achieved between having long enough testing intervals in order to reduce practice effects and not having them too far apart as to miss early critical changes. Generally, six month intervals are considered the optimum, with more frequent testing for infants and children who are symptomatic.

The value of such extensive investigations of children and their families who are already under great stress is frequently questioned by many professionals who feel that any findings result in limited positive intervention and contribute little by way of improved quality of care in the long term. However, in the case of paediatric AIDS and HIV infection, the value of systematic assessment can be argued on a number of grounds.

On a global basis, any systematically collected body of data which directly relates to the process of this illness will add to our understanding and may ultimately direct treatment and care in a more beneficial way.

- Much information at the moment is based on retrospective data and is therefore biased to those who are symptomatic. Systematic assessment on infected but non-symptomatic children will contribute useful information

on the natural history of HIV infection in children.
- Regular assessments may help identify the prevalence of neurologic signs and symptoms and developmental delay in infected children.
- Regular assessments may help identify the nature of such impairment and how children are affected at different ages and stages in the disease process.
- The type of neurological effects are also believed to be related to the child's age or point of development at which HIV infection occurs. This again could be clarified if children are regularly and reliably assessed.
- Such assessments can provide additional information and help in the evaluation of drug trials and other aspects of medical intervention.
- Accurate planning for future service provision will require accurate knowledge about the future needs of these children. This will be particularly important where improved medical intervention may lead to increased life expectancy but perhaps with continued deterioration, thus resulting in a new generation of children with special educational, health and social needs. There are implications here not only for medical services but also paramedical services such as speech therapists, physiotherapists, psychologists and occupational therapists who may be providing the bulk of remedial help and support.

On an individual basis, early and repeated neurological assessment can provide a useful monitor of how the child is progressing through his or her illness and treatment in a number of ways.

- Signs of neurological impairment and developmental delay can be picked up early.
- The nature of the impairment can be defined clearly.
- Additions or changes to medical intervention can be monitored to see their effect on the identified problems.
- Where neurological impairment is persistent through treatment, early and individualised remedial help can be provided.

There are a number of ways in which such assessments can clearly also be of benefit to the family as a whole.

- Worried parents and carers can be reassured that their child is developing normally, if this is indeed the case.
- Parents and carers can be shown that treatment is facilitating recovery of lost function even if this progress is slow and not easy to observe directly.
- Where there are signs of persistent neurological deterioration, parents and carers can be key helpers in any appropriate remedial techniques. In this way they may feel empowered and useful in a situation where they otherwise feel completely powerless and helpless.

If neuropsychological assessments are to be helpful both to our understanding of the effects of HIV infection on the developing central nervous system and to the life of the individual child who is infected, there are however a number of cautionary steps which need to be taken.

The tests used should be chosen carefully and must be reliable and valid. Care also needs to be taken to distinguish and identify between impairment due to HIV infection and that due to anxiety, repeated illness and perhaps hospitalisation, medication, missed schooling, failure to thrive, parental intravenous drug misuse and other physical and social factors which may bias the results and confuse the overall picture.

A further point to be noted is that while the numbers of infected children at any one treatment centre are small, wider knowledge and general understanding of paediatric HIV infection will only be gained if different centres seek to collaborate and use mutually compatible assessment procedures and techniques.

References

1. Brouwers, P., Belman, A., Epstein, L. (1990). Central nervous system involvement: manifestations and evaluation. In Pizzo, P. A., Wilfert, C. M. (eds), *Paediatric AIDS: The Challenge of HIV Infection in Infants, Children and Adolescents*. Williams and Wilkins, Baltimore.
2. Belman, A.L., Ultmann, M.H., Horoupian, D. *et al.* (1985). Neurological complications in infants and children with acquired immune deficiency syndrome. *Annals of Neurology*, **18(5)**, 560–6.
3. Belman, A.L., Diamond, G., Dickson, D. *et al.* (1988). Paediatric acquired immunodeficiency syndrome. *ADJC*, **142**, 29–35.
4. Epstein, L.G., Sharer, L.R., Joshi, V.V. *et al.* (1985). Progressive encephalopathy in children with acquired immune deficiency syndrome. *Annals of Neurology*, **17**, 488–96.
5. Epstein, L.G., Sharer, L.R., Oleske, J.M. *et al.* (1989). Neurologic manifestations of human immunodeficiency virus infection in children. *Journal of Paediatrics*, **1144**, 1–30.
6. European Collaborative Study (1990). Neurologic signs in young children with HIV infection. *Journal of Paediatric Infectious Disease*, **9**, 402–6.

11 Aspects of psychological support for families and children affected by HIV

Jim Kuykendall

I wish to dedicate this chapter to Steven – the first young man I had the privilege to support in his dying, and to the many children and young people together with their families and partners who have given me so much through their lives and their deaths.

The family as the patient

Paediatric philosophy suggests that the entire family is the patient. This maxim could not be more true than when caring for children and adolescents with HIV disease. HIV not only compromises the child's immune system, but challenges the psychological immunity and the integrity of the entire family unit. Children with HIV can become isolated and alone in their illness, and siblings can be stigmatised by society and overprotected (or neglected) by their parents. Individual family members can become too overwhelmed by their own issues with regard to HIV to continue functioning effectively as part of the family. The whole family can be overcome with despair as it considers the issues and difficulties of living with uncertainty, isolation, death and possible multiple loss. HIV can threaten the very continuance of the family – the very ability to live with AIDS and all its ramifications. As HIV breaks down the immune system within the individual, it lays the family open to a host of psychological 'opportunistic infections' such as self-recrimination and guilt, prejudice, bigotry, harrassment at work and school to name but a few. Families are also pushed into dilemmas concerning the 'protection of rights' and the 'best interest' of their child – within a society that, in 'demanding to know', discriminates against their child. AIDS is a family disease.

A developmental approach

To be able to address these family needs, caregivers need to recognise that all illness changes according to the developmental issues being negotiated at that time by the HIV-infected child/adolescent and by the siblings of the child. As such, caregivers require a working knowledge of normal child and adolescent development in order to understand how chronic life-threatening illness impinges upon these developmental issues. Only through such understanding can patients be supported *to live* with AIDS rather than solely *to die* from AIDS. The following cases illustrate the types of developmental issues raised.

Tim is a very bright 14-year-old boy with haemophilia and HIV infection. Tim's parents knew that he had HIV infection but did not wish Tim to know this. Being very aware that some Factor VIII had been contaminated, Tim argued with his parents for several months, insisting that he had the right to be tested so that he could know his HIV status. After family pre-test counselling his parents reluctantly agreed.

For Tim, being HIV infected focussed around the issue of peer acceptance. He desperately needed to know that he could tell his friends and would still belong; that he would still be approved of, and seen as the same person by his peers. Whilst counselling could not reassure him of that, it did provide a forum to explore the issue of whether he really needed to tell them and why, as well as what it would mean if he was openly rejected by them. Other issues for Tim included self-identity, sexuality and his ability to marry and have children. Miller and Bor[1] have found the question about marriage and having children very common among teenagers.

Developmentally, adolescents of Tim's age still think of themselves as invincible and indestructible, and as such it did not appear to the staff that Tim has any concerns about illness and dying.

Tim's father's immediate question however was about how long Tim had to live. His mother's concern was about if, when and what to tell Tim's four- and seven-year-old sisters. Over time, both parents began to grapple with the loss of the future that they had felt Factor VIII had secured for them.

Five-year-old Lucy was infected with HIV but asymptomatic. Her parents had little support outside the hospital and requested strict confidentiality about their situation. Visits to the hospital were a difficult experience for the family, as they reminded Lucy's parents of the potential threat of illness.

For Lucy's parents their concerns were if and what to tell their young daughter and if and what to tell the teachers at the school she attended. They were also trying to treat Lucy as normally as possible, without over protecting her at a time when the issue of Lucy's independence was being attempted.

Sixteen-year-old Martin experienced sexual and emotional isolation as he attempted to come to terms with his newly discovered homosexual identity as well as being HIV positive. Martin felt that there was no one whom he could trust with this discovery, let alone reveal his HIV status to. As he felt that intimacy must lead to rejection he became celibate, isolated and withdrawn.

Approaches used by caregivers need to be as creative and diversified as their patients. For Lucy, communicating through play assisted her to work through some of the fantasies and the misperceptions that she had for why she was regularly attending hospital. Likewise, Tim's younger sisters were supported through play therapy to express their feelings of desertion and impotence as the family became more and more involved with Tim.

Support for the family

Tim's parents found great support with the staff in the Haemophilia Centre that had always had a long caring relationship with the family. Other parents however, are not so fortunate.

Barbara Peabody, an American mother was distressed when her son was diagnosed with AIDS and she was subsequently abandoned by all her work colleagues and friends. She became determined that other parents would not experience this intense rejection and desertion, and created a network of support groups for parents throughout the United States. An organisation was created to help parents to contact and gain support from other parents in the same situation.

In the United Kingdom, Positively Women, Body Positive, Terrence Higgins Trust, London Lighthouse, Mildmay Mission Hospital, Landmark, and other statutory and non-statutory organisations are beginning to respond to and create support systems and groups available for parents, or who welcome parents and/or their children who have HIV infection (see Appendix).

Some parents find great difficulty in approaching organisations that were initially created to address the needs of a specially targeted group, for example injecting drug users or gay people. Hence many parents still feel isolated. Parents who are injecting drug users can feel cut off from society, with feelings of isolation and rejection, even before their or their child's status is known.

This stark reality becomes everymore distressing as we realise that many times there may be several individuals within the family who have HIV infection with possibly two or more individuals ill at the same time.

Sixteen-year-old Martin (see p. 147) benefited through discussions of safer sex. He was scared of infecting others and lacked the social skill necessary to negotiate safer sex with a potential partner. His Health Adviser was able to give him factual information about transmission and prevention as well as referring him for therapy, thus enabling him to work through intense guilt, embarrassment and confusion and to come to terms with his homosexuality.

In working with clients, consideration is given to whether any individual, family, group or marital therapy might be appropriate. For Martin, it was obvious that individual therapy afforded him the complete confidentiality, time and space to disclose his feelings and personal thoughts in privacy. Martin was able to build up a close and trusting relationship with his counsellor and challenge some of his issues around intimacy leading to rejection. Five months into therapy his counsellor was able to introduce Martin to another adolescent who had successfully negotiated forming a meaningful relationship after being diagnosed as HIV-positive.

During a difficult period for Tim's parents (see p. 147) they requested individual sessions so that they could explore a split that they felt widening between them since Tim's HIV diagnosis. Several sessions proved useful but it was also appreciated that this choice of therapeutic arena, while initially beneficial, mirrored their split. Although counselling began individually as had been requested, it was then possible to move them into therapy together. Resistance to this shift was acknowledged and this insight enabled them to address some of their obstacles.

It has been found that group psychotherapy can meet the special needs of some clients with HIV disease where indicated. El-Mallakh and El-Mallakh[2] have reported that 'people who have become socially isolated and estranged from family and community because of AIDS can find support and sympathetic contact in a person with AIDS (PWA) support group'. In identifying the complex factors that go into the making of a successful group, Yalom[3] listed the following problems:

- universality
- imparting of information
- instillation of hope
- family re-enactment
- group cohesiveness and
- catharsis.

El-Mallakh and El-Mallakh[2] state that people with AIDS benefit from several of Yalom's factors.

Universality can impart the feeling that the group member is not alone – others share his dilemmas and concerns. Information exchange occurs when knowledge regarding HIV disease is shared. Family re-enactment can occur if the group provides the familiar support that is not otherwise received. Likewise, group cohesion may provide a feeling of acceptance and belonging to group members. This acceptance may encourage catharsis.

Whatever the approach Sider and Clements[4] state 'that the choice of psychotherapeutic modality is not only a matter of personal preference or efficacy of technique, it is also a matter of ethics'.

As there are many other co-factors in this decision-making, I refer the interested reader to the indications and contra-indications for individual therapy discussed in Dryden[5].

Most importantly care-givers must not prevent people (whether young or old) from using their own coping strategies. HIV already takes enough away. Those with HIV or AIDS are, at times, so overwhelmed by a new diagnosis or by the presentation of a new or repeated opportunistic infection that they forget how they have coped with the other large issues in their life. This applies to both children and adults. Individuals are able to create coping strategies contingent upon the opportunity and ability to create past problem solving skills, as well as upon chronological and maturational development. This includes children with learning difficulties. Granted they may want and need to hand over the decision-making and control at times (for example during an acute episode of illness, during a confused mental state, or simply because they traditionally need to believe that the care giver 'knows best'), but this can readily feed into a paternalistic health care system that removes individual's autonomy under the guise of 'don't worry or fret about it, we know what is best for you'.

In a study of biomedical ethics, the principles of autonomy and beneficence consider the possibility that in actual fact we might not know, and certainly in isolation of the client might not be able to know, what is in the client's best interest. These principles invite care-givers to work alongside and with clients and/or patients, so that they can achieve a better understanding of any situation and what all the available options are at that time. This includes non-consent to treatment and care. Obviously this is over-simplified, and readers will be able to identify situations and impediments to this.

Nevertheless, autonomy and benificence are principles that caregivers often give lip service to as being essential to clients without having thought through mechanisms to implement them. With a disease where loss of dignity, control, body image, independence, certainty and perhaps loss of some established support systems are often seen, caregivers have a strong obligation to allow clients/patients (whether parents or the children) to become as autonomous as they can.

A review with the parent may help to refocus and reassess what supports already exist within/for them and their child/children. The following approach has been found to be of value.

- Ask the individual what they personally do for themselves that help and support them during difficult times. Responses might include yoga, autogenic breathing exercise, meditation, visualisation, walking ... Check if these will still be possible.
- Ask what external supports exist for the individual. This could include the babysitter who relieves the parents for a couple of hours a week, the vicar's visit, contact with neighbours and relatives ... Check if these supports are still there. Fear and prejudice around HIV can destroy previously staunch support systems.
- Ask what statutory and or voluntary involvement exists. This might include buddies, a home help, meals on wheels, the district nurse, the GP, the community psychiatric nurse, the aromatherapist among others. (A 'buddy' is a befriender – a volunteer helper working with specialist agencies in the field of HIV/AIDS.)
- Plot this onto a visual chart with the client and then determine if he or she already feels well supported – or over supported – and if not, what they feel their needs still are. This enables the caregiver to not only share what they can proffer but to find out what/where the gaps might be and refer accordingly.

[Obviously some of these coping strategies will not be relevant to young children. However, appropriate coping mechanisms for them can be explored as well, when necessary. Ed.]

Coping through play

In the past, children's play has been considered by some to be a 'superfluous activity', an activity only important as it allowed the child a release of excess energy. However, experience suggests that play can offer and effect much more – play is essential as a problem solving approach into childhood; play is fun, exploratory and relieves boredom and it maintains and promotes normal development. There is no difference between play and the work of the child; play is the best use of the child's time.

The sick child, however, is certainly at a disadvantage for maintaining play. Any illness that challenges the child's mobility and desire to involve him or herself in play can threaten a child's sense of worth and self concept. Children with chronic illness are at high emotional and social risk. Children with HIV, especially older children who have an understanding of the illness, can present as withdrawn, anxious or non-communicative and suicidal.

Play activities that are short term, easily achievable and that bolster the child's sense of worth allow a sense of mastery. Play therapy allows a child to confront distressing issues surrounding illness in a safe and familiar environment.

Five-year-old Lucy (see p. 147), already in hospital one month, walked up to the Wendy house and slammed the door saying 'Lucy doesn't live here anymore'. The hospital play specialist went into the Wendy house and asked Lucy to knock again. This time she was told how much she was missed at home and how quickly everyone wanted her to get better and return home. Lucy then appeared happier and joined in the group cooking activity.

Play allows a child to express negative feelings in an acceptable, safe and indirect way.

> Tim's four-year-old sister, Mary (see p. 147), released considerable anger through the use of animal and finger puppets. The puppet yelled at the doll who didn't care about her anymore and who spent all her time with Tim.

Through therapeutic play Mary was able to work through some of her feelings towards Tim and her parents. Research by Spinetta and Spinetta[6] showed that siblings fared worse in overall adjustment and worse than both parents and patient during times of crisis.

Drawing and painting can provide a ready medium for expression. Children graphically portray their feelings of anger, depression, isolation and impotency in relation to catastrophic illness and other life traumas. Visualisation and art therapy can be used to help children express needs and mobilise resources for a meaningful life. The value of imagery in working with children and adolescents with HIV disease is that it can be used not only as a diversion from unpleasant experiences but assist many of these non-communicative, withdrawn children to communicate their feelings through stories. Children and adolescents too helpless to move from their beds can explore future plans and realise goals in symbolic form therapy, experiencing some of the independence and creativity denied them through their illness. For children who have withdrawn into apathy and helplessness, the expression of wishes and desires and the exercise of independence through imagery may, by themselves, create new excitement and interest.

A checklist for caregivers

When preparing a child or sibling to look at issues surrounding HIV disease, caregivers need to take into account and check out some straightforward practical points. The experience of having a patient or sibling with HIV disease is effected by many factors. The following are a few examples of issues that may (or may not) need addressing.

i   Who in the family has HIV disease, and/or the number of individuals infected with HIV, while recognising that all family members are affected by it. (Some members may not be aware of an HIV diagnosis within the family.)

ii The family and child's knowledge base, and understanding of HIV disease.

iii An appreciation of the child's and family's views and feelings about HIV disease.

iv The cultural and religious backgrounds of families with HIV disease. (A recent tour throughout the Middle East reminded the author of just how difficult or inappropriate it is for some individuals and cultures to talk openly about sexual issues and bereavement difficulties. Also how strained family relationships can become as caregivers attempt to create a parity among family members where it would not otherwise exist.) Understanding cultural differences allows the creation of approaches optimal towards that culture.

Reactions to bad news

There is a range of possible reactions that any one individual child or adult may or may not manifest. For many individuals shock, denial and an inability to hear or comprehend may serve as a first line of defence. During this period, emotional and physical numbness and withdrawal may result. Over time, some children show marked regression, infantile behaviour and relinquish developmental milestones already attained. Others, however, may intellectualise, or feel intense anger or profound sadness. Some other adolescents and adults may feel relief at finally having a diagnosis of the expected illness at the end of a long period of expectation. Additionally, younger children especially, who cannot understand some of the implications of receiving an HIV or AIDS diagnosis, may be very able to deal with the bad news, yet through the principle of contagion and contamination absorb, internalise and act out the feelings of parents and significant others, including staff. This emphasises the importance of monitoring the whole family unit as well as supporting the staff on an ongoing basis. Children, as patients, many times become a 'sponge' for the displaced feelings around them. It is then imperative to appreciate that not only may a child feel guilty for being diagnosed HIV positive or for having AIDS, because many children are told by adults that whatever happens 'is all their fault', but that the child may absorb some of the parents guilt for transmitting HIV or for giving contaminated blood or blood products to the child.

The loss of the sense of security and the uncertainty that many adults experience are very powerful developmental issues that still need to be negotiated by all children, whether the patient or his or her siblings. In Maslow's hierarchy of needs model, children always need to be reassured that their first level needs will continue to be met, i.e. food, shelter, being looked after etc. It is not coincidental that children, after the death of a parent/ guardian, will ask 'who will look after them?' This egocentric question needs to be satisfied before it is at all possible for children to regain some sense of security. This poses quite a dilemma in families where multiples of individuals may be infected with HIV, and where the very continuance of the family unit is threatened. Caregivers need to be very aware of this as they plan support systems for the family. Some of the destabilising effects may be acted out behaviourally in schools or at home – giving clues to caregivers as to how children are coping. Reactions of decreased self-esteem, loss of identity, personal control and fear have also been reported. Children will be affected according to how adults are able to negotiate these issues around HIV disease and AIDS. General practitioners, health visitors, school nurses, teachers, social workers and all other community based and hospital staff need to ascertain how both the adult and child members of the family are coping. In so doing, caregivers can provide the support that will help reduce adult contagion and help the child focus and process issues in ways appropriate to the child.

A new disease for the child and family

After time, tests, treatments and disease can become routine to caregivers. However, to children, investigations, tests, treatments and diseases are not routine and the child needs to be prepared for them. This preparation can help in replacing any fantasies, misperceptions and misconceptions with reality, and can help to either desensitise fears or create appropriate coping strategies. Whether the child is undergoing a drug trial, having treatment or a check-up, he or she has entered a totally new world. What may be routine protocol for the caregiver may be unfamiliar and frightening to children.

The Platt Report[7] found that illness and hospitalisation can prove very destabilising to the psychological welfare of the child, as he or she is exposed to new sights, sounds, smells, people and routines, all in a new environment. The structures that have made the child safe and contained are replaced by ever changing 'routines' and expectations. The established safe structures themselves may change as other individuals within the family unit become infected and/or affected by HIV disease.

Messages around coping

Any caregiver who is concerned about any members of a family with HIV, should discuss this concern *both* with the appropriate adult members of the family and with relevant staff. It will not be helpful to the family if a psychiatric or psychological referral of the child is made without the parents knowledge and consent. Care has to be taken when offering support – there may be a need for psychological or psychiatric intervention, but this must be arranged with discretion. Counselling and therapeutic support for families may be appropriate and offered when necessary. It is known for adults in a family affected by HIV to think and speak of suicide, and these feelings should be greatly explored and appropriately addressed by experienced staff. It is important to emphasise the need for skilled help to be offered to families who are overwhelmed by shock and anxiety when confronted with the many difficulties that HIV encompasses. However, there are many families who cope and need no extra help other than the knowledge that support is available when it is necessary. Some may be using the coping strategy of denial – this is a common way of managing, and it would be inappropriate and inadvisable for unskilled care givers to destroy this form of coping mechanism.

Young people with HIV disease should be encouraged not to be ashamed or afraid of who they are and what they have, and not to be ashamed or afraid of the way they feel or think. They may need reassurance that most people with a new diagnosis of HIV and/or AIDS feel many different emotions and that they are not alone in this – it is quite usual to feel such emotions in these circumstances. In listening to, valuing and accepting these feelings, the care giver will give the person permission to begin working through this painful and difficult stage of their life.

It is important that children and young people with HIV and AIDS recognise that, no matter what they read or who they talk to, each person is different. An individual with HIV is not a number, and how an individual's body reacts to treatment may be different from other people's reactions. Children must have confidence in themselves and in the treatment they will be having.

By enabling clients to explore their worst fears early on, there is no taboo that they cannot share with the caregiver as time goes on. People with HIV and/or AIDS should be told to give themselves time to adjust to physical changes, and that it is understandable and necessary to mourn and feel those changes. They should be reassured that the qualities that other people like – their sense of humour, their kindness, their courage – will not go away.

The caregiver can ask the patient to help in finding the correct support and treatment that will help them *live with* AIDS.

Letting go – the need for closure

> And the time has come for me to be gone
> I have fought the good fight to the end
> I have run the race to the finish
> Ecclesiastes

Children, like adults, need the opportunity to complete their own unfinished business.

> Mark, a six-year-old dying of leukaemia, told staff that he would not be seeing them when they returned from the Christmas holidays in a fortnight's time. I needed to clarify with him what he meant. Matter of factly he said: 'I'm going to be dead, of course'. After letting him know how sad I would be not to be seeing him in January, I wondered if there was any way that I could help him with things that he still needed to do. Mark's face brightened and he said that he wanted to give away his baseball and football caps. As there were 18 caps in his collection, I dutifully sat down and asked who was to receive what. 'Parents to receive two each, brothers and sisters one each, best friend three, other friends one and counsellor one'. The final cap he wanted to wear when he died. His will had been recorded and was executed one week later.

The requests are as varied as each unique child who makes them. They are usually painful for staff and family to hear, for by acknowledging the request we acknowledge the reality.

Tim, the 14-year-old with HIV (see p. 147) needed to visit his school and friends one last time before returning home to die. Unable to walk he was wheeled to the gym, locker room and home room where he touched all the people and the objects that were special to him. This very poignant scene was very difficult for his friends who needed a lot of support in order to help Tim and themselves to say goodbye.

As so often happens 'closure' requests are blocked by loved ones who need to deny its meaning.

> Ten-year-old Simon insisted that he return home for one last time. Within 24 hours, he had given away his guitar to his best friend, cars to his younger brother and computer video to his older brother. It was his older brother Michael who chided Simon that within a few days he would be feeling much better and would feel very stupid having given everything away. Simon, strong within himself, ignored this remark and said: 'You know Mike, if heaven is as good a place as it is cracked up to be, I'll have an even better computer there'.

Many young people, however, internalise adult messages like 'Don't be silly, of course you are getting better', 'What a morbid way to talk', 'Pull yourself together and have a cup of tea' and 'You will be fit in no time at all'. These messages reinforce the idea of not facing death. The child, family members and staff become isolated from each other at the most central time of their lives.

With a catastrophic diagnosis, people do need to protect themselves at least some of the time. This understandably disallows parents from being able to admit and to say to children many of the things that they cannot yet admit and say to themselves. However, in addition to this, the prejudice, fears and bigotries of family members, neighbours and society as a whole may disallow young clients from their closure. Clients have been prevented from returning to secondary school or college, and a young girl was unable to return to her art class and Saturday club. Instead of support, these clients were met with rejection, desertion and isolation. They became lone and shameful mourners of their fate.

However, for Tim (p. 147), it was different. When he lapsed into his unconsciousness he was surrounded by his family and friends. He continued floating in and out of consciousness and was reassured by their voices. His mate held his hand and spoke of a soccer game that they had both played together. His mother stroked his hair – and he died.

An example of one form of 'letting go' is the AIDS Memorial Quilt which was designed and sewn together to commemorate the life of individuals who have died from AIDS. The panels have been created by lovers, families, friends, caregivers and individuals with HIV disease. The Quilt now almost 12 000 individual panels of $3' \times 6'$, with more than 20 000 names on it. Celebrity names like Rock Hudson and Liberace appear next to not so well known names and there are blank panels for visitors to the Quilt to record names. The Quilt was first displayed on 11 October 1987 in front of the US Capital in Washington DC where it covered a space larger than two football fields. It has returned to Washington DC each October and parts of it has toured major American and Canadian cities. Quilts are now being made in various cities around the world.

A quilt provides a way to grieve and a way to remember. It transforms AIDS from a virus to human faces with individual stories. Each panel talks of courage, fear, anger but mostly of love. It portrays people who worked and played, who laughed and cried, who lived and died and who now are remembered. A quilt such as this also provides an opportunity for children to remember their parent or sibling. In making a quilt panel the child can be allowed personal expression of his or her feelings. [An alternative would be in encouraging the child to create a picture in memory of the person who has died. Ed.]

Bereavement – a long term process

Bereavement is both a cognitive and an emotive long term process. A process through which individuals mourn not only the loss of the individual whom they love but also the loss of all those things, events and places that were special to the person who died and the survivors who are left behind. Bereavement is also the mourning of the part of themselves that dies with the loved person's death – the dying person may have called the survivor by a special name and, with the person's death, one is no longer called by that name. In fact, individuals may resent being called that special name by others as it was reserved between them and their loved one.

Children and bereavement

Even very young children have perceptions regarding death and dying, and they too have a bereavement process which is facilitated or hindered by adults. This is understandable, as it may be difficult for adults to imagine children entering into grief work as they watch the dead child's siblings returning home from the funeral, change their clothes and run out to play. Children cannot consciously hold onto and tolerate feelings such as sadness, depression and anger in the same way that adults are able to. For their needs, as well as for fulfilling adult needs (big boys don't cry; stiff upper lip, etc.) children learn rapidly to respond in expected ways. Some children are disallowed entry into or fixated within their bereavement. Some manifest this in changed behaviour patterns (picking more fights, becoming the loner, overcompensatory action, etc.). Others will repress it and enter into a benign or quiescent phase – only to manifest symptoms later in life. Caregivers must, however, be very clear that one powerful maxim in bereavement counselling applies to both children and adults. Bereavement that is not processed is either represssed or acted out. If acted out it can be either behaviourally, somatically or psychosomatically manifested. Adults need to allow children (as well as other adults for that matter) to talk about and feel the loss. Such permission allows children, both in the present and in the future, to come back and ask more questions about the death and share that they too, like their parents, feel sad, angry or guilty. Social, intellectual and emotional inclusion throughout the illness and after death facilitates the child's bereavement process. For example, the immediate replacement of a dead pet, while protecting both the child and the adult, does not allow the child the opportunity to create coping strategies and skills to deal with the issues that surround the death. The immediate return to normal for the childrens' sake after the death of a sibling can be even more problem-laden. Children can misinterpret their parents as callous and as parents who truly did not love the dead child. Instead of parents protecting the children from their own grief, they can isolate the child with their own unacknowledged grief, and additionally give the opportunity for misconceptions and fantasies around the life and death of the dead child.

> Eight-year-old Susie presented for therapy after continued disruptive behaviour began in school shortly after the death of her 13-year-old sister Terry (who had died in a road traffic accident). Her behaviour was a dramatic change from the affable and co-operative person that everyone knew.

It was discovered that Susie's mother, in trying to shield her daughter from her own intense pain, always put on a cheerful face for her daughter. The eight year old, however, misinterpreted her mother's cheerfulness. She thought that her mother had already forgotten Terry and felt that she may never have loved her. Susie's fear then became 'did her mother really love Susie?' This fantasy and fear of additional loss and rejection from her mother both scared her and made her furious. At eight years of age she did not know how to deal with these thoughts and feelings, and subsequently acted them out.

A very different acting out behaviour is one of over-compensation in which the sibling becomes the 'ideal' child – the perfect child at school or home or both. Extended inability to concentrate in school work or on other tasks can also indicate breavement problems.

In any situation where multiple loss occurs, complications in the bereavement process becomes even more possible. Families that include several individuals with HIV infection may be both in anticipatory grief as well as in bereavement for a member who has already died. Each individual can be at a different stage in their own bereavement process leaving other members to feel alone or isolated in their own grief. Many families, communities and care givers can become locked in the bereavement process for years. Feelings of being totally overwhelmed, despair, frustration and intense anger amongst others need to be vented in ways appropriate to each individual. Some defence mechanisms may be further developed – intellectualisation, denial, avoidance, rationalisation are very often employed by caregivers, especially in the absence of support for these particular caregivers.

The staff: an issue of non-support

In HIV work staff compare with siblings as being the most neglected and least supported group. Historically, staff neglect might evolve from nursing and medical schools that train their students 'to cope with everything' no matter how horrendous the situation. Subsequently, in creating such a Nietzschean philosophy of superman and superwoman, which suggests that doctors and nurses can do everything, individual staff find it difficult in accepting support, even when it is proffered.

Recent studies have considered the personality types of individuals who become caregivers. Although findings show multifactorial reasons, and more research is needed, one of the conclusions might suggest that people labelled as caregivers find more comfort and control in giving care than in receiving it. This can pose serious problems for staff who, for example in treating children with Factor VIII so that they could lead 'normal' lives, are now watching these same children become gravely ill and die. Many staff in these situations report feelings of guilt, inadequacy and helplessness. Likewise, staff who came into Paediatric or into STD/GUM clinics to care for clients with acute illnesses amenable to present day therapies are feeling overwhelmed and frustrated by a disease that is not acute, that is ultimately not amenable to current treatments and that has replaced cancer for its degree of stigma and abhorrence.

Staff do indeed need support and this can be given in several ways. As with clients, it is important not to deskill staff, but first to check with them what supports already exist and how adequate these support systems are for them.

Staff support through education

Health care organisations need to create programmes or 'menus' for support from which staff can choose 'à la carte' those items most suitable for them. For example, staff commencing employment in a health authority could attend an HIV Orientation Day and, once in post, attend speciality focus days and update days.

Focus days could address such areas as HIV and drug use, paediatric HIV, neurological issues and HIV, counselling and HIV. Update days present the latest findings to staff regarding HIV issues. Additionally, courses on 'The care and management of individuals with HIV infection' could be offered annually. Such programmes of, for example, 12–17 days, could proffer a comprehensive look into all aspects of HIV disease, from epidemiology and tramission through to ethical issues, bereavement and loss, sexuality, women's issues about HIV, drug use and HIV and health education, exploring issues of clients/patients with HIV both in the hospital and community setting. Workshops also enable staff to improve and enlarge their communication and counselling skills. All training and updating of knowledge about HIV and AIDS should adopt a multidiscplinary approach within the hospital and transdisciplinary between community and hospitals.

Staff support by other means

On the emotional menu stress awareness and stress reduction workshops should be offered by the employing authority and individual staff counselling and staff support groups facilitated. When patients with HIV disease die, ward staff may be invited to attend a 5–10 minute session to enable staff to say whatever it is that they need to about the person who has just died. This can be very beneficial in acting as a catalyst for the caregivers own bereavement process. Finally, keeping the cardex intact for 24 hours after the person's death enables oncoming staff the opportunity to officially acknowledge and discuss the person's death – rather than only being able to talk about the person who has already taken their bed.

There is much to gain through staff being able to keep in touch with each other. This enables them to benefit from sharing up-to-date information, and peer group support. This can be made possible through local and national groups as well as through Conferences and Study days.

In conclusion, it is important to reiterate that HIV is a family disease. The family needs appropriate support in order for discordance to be avoided. For any group of people faced with all the difficulties that HIV and AIDS manifests, caregivers will need to continually monitor the family and offer help in preparing for an uncertain future. As yet there are no models of psychological care for this family situation, because there are endless combinations of psychological, social and physical problems to be confronted, together with a health care system that is not fully integrating care for parents and their children. However families with HIV will feel valued if there is a caregiver who is able to attend and listen in a non-judgemental way – giving the family time and space to explore their feelings.

References

1. Miller, R., Bor, R. (1990). Psychological and socio-medical aspects of AIDS/HIV. *AIDS Care*, **3(1)**.
2. El-Mallakh and El-Mallakh (1984). Therapeutic Arenas. In *Individual Therapy in Britain*, W. Dryden (ed.), Open University Press, Milton Keynes.
3. Yalom, I. D. (1975). *The Theory and Practice of Group Psychotherapy*, second edition. Basic Books, New York.
4. Sider, R. C., Clements, C. (1982). Family or individual therapy. The ethics of modality choice. *American Journal of Psychiatry*, **139(11)**, 1455–9.
5. Dryden, W. (1984). Therapeutic Arenas. In *Individual Therapy in Britain*, W. Dryden (ed.), Open University Press, Milton Keynes.
6. Spinetta, J., Spinetta, P. (1981). *Living with Childhood Cancer*, St Louis, Mosby.
7. Ministry of Health (1959). *The Welfare of Children in Hospital*. Report of Central Health Services Council Chairman: Sir Harry Platt. HMSO, London.

Further reading

Kuykendall, J. W. (1988). Play Therapy. In *The Supportive Care of the Child with Cancer*, A. Oakhill (ed.), Wright, London.

Kuykendall, J. W. (1989). Death of a Child – The Worst Kept Secret Around. In *Death, Dying and Bereavement*, L. Sherr (ed.), Blackwell Scientific Publications, Oxford.

Miller, R., Goldman, E. *et al.* (1989). AIDS and children: some of the issues in haemophilia care and how to address them. *AIDS Care*, **1(1)**, 59–65.

Pizzi, M. (1990). The role of occupational therapy in the multidisciplinary care of children with HIV infection. *Paediatric AIDS and HIV Infection: Fetus to Adolescence*, **1(3)**, 11–15.

Sherr, L. (1989). A guide for workers dealing with children. In *Death, Dying and Bereavement*, L. Sherr (ed.), Blackwell Scientific Publications, Oxford.

Waterbury, M. (1990). Counselling the HIV infected adolescent. *Paediatric AIDS and HIV Infection: Fetus to Adolescent*, **1(2)**, 18–20.

12 Infection control

Susan Macqueen

Providing a safe environment is a fundamental role for all health care workers in any setting – whether in hospital, at home or in the community. Since families with children may have fears of cross-infection, this chapter provides a background of information enabling all those involved to be aware of the advantages of reliable infection control. Wherever appropriate all carers, including parents, may need to be aware of the simple measures required in order to avoid both unnecessary fears and the risk of infection. If all care providers are aware of and utilise infection control guidelines this will provide:

- reassurance to personal safety
- appropriate and not excessive use of isolation precautions
- security, thus reducing the risk of psychological isolation
- a reduction in the risk of spreading infection.

The general lack of knowledge of microbiology, virology and infectious diseases reinforces the fear of the unknown. Therefore it is the responsibility of all health care providers to seek information that will enable them to care with confidence for all those with HIV infection.

Health Authorities have a legal obligation under the Health and Safety at Work Act (1974) to ensure that all employees are appropriately trained and proficient in the procedures necessary for working safely. Equally, every employee has a duty to take reasonable care of the health and safety of him or herself and other persons who may be affected by his or her acts or omissions at work.

Furthermore, employers are required by the Control of Substances Hazardous to Health (COSHH) regulations (1988), enforced on 1st October 1989, to review regularly every procedure carried out by their employees which involved contact with substances hazardous to health. These substances include micro-organisms.

Universal precautions

Since 1983, health-care workers in the USA have been encouraged to use 'universal precautions'. As it is often impossible to know whether an individual has been infected with HIV (or other blood-borne infections such as hepatitis B), policies and practices that reduce health-care workers' exposure to blood and body fluids from all patients should be developed[1]. These principles should be implemented both in hospitals, in the community, and schools and playgroups, etc., where child health care is provided, and should apply to all those involved including the child's family and relatives.

The following guidelines are based on the recommendations from the

Expert Advisory Group on AIDS from the Department of Health (UK), together with the Technical Panel on Infections within Hospitals of the American Hospital Association with assistance from the Centre of Disease Control in Atlanta, USA.

Health care staff carrying out clinical and non-clinical procedures for children and adults should at all times have due regard to written policies produced by their employing authority. Further advice and information may be sought from the local Infection Control Nurse, the Infection Control Officer or the Consultant Microbiologist or Virologist, where appropriate.

Transmission of HIV infection

HIV has been isolated from blood, semen, vaginal secretions, saliva, tears, urine, breastmilk, cerebro-spinal, synovial and amniotic fluids. However, only the following have been implicated in the transmission of the infection:

- blood
- blood products
- semen
- vaginal secretions
- donor organs and tissues
- breastmilk (see Chapters 1, 6 and 7).

To date, there has been no evidence of faecal-oral or airborne spread of HIV, nor spread from saliva. It is possible for the virus to be transmitted across intact mucous membrane or conjunctiva, but in common with hepatitis B, it appears improbable that HIV could penetrate intact skin. (See also Chapter 1.)

In practice, clinical procedures which involve body fluids listed in Table 12.1 usually involve potential contact with blood. Therefore *all* reference to blood in the context of HIV transmission should be taken to include all the body fluids mentioned below.

Table 12.1 Body fluids which should be handled with the same precautions as those taken with blood and all blood products

Cerebro-spinal fluid (CSF)	Semen
Blood products	Vaginal secretions
Peritoneal fluid	Any other body fluid containing visible
Pleural fluid	blood
Pericardial fluid	Saliva in association with dentistry
Synovial fluid	Unfixed tissues and organs
Amniotic fluid	

Avoiding transmission of infection

The main principles in avoiding person-to-person transmission of HIV and other blood-borne pathogens are to:

- assess the task risk factors involved
- wear appropriate protective clothing for exposure to 'high risk' body fluids (see above)
- avoid sharps and needlestick injuries
- maintain a high standard of hygiene
- implement effective training programmes for all health care workers.

Assess the task risk factors involved

The following framework is suggested for assessing the risk of clinical work practices in the context of transmission of blood-borne pathogens in the area of paediatric care[2].

High risk category

The full range of protective clothing should be worn where exposure to uncontrolled bleeding or splattering is high, for example, during surgical and obstetric procedures. The level of precautions should generally include the use of the following:

- gloves
- water repellent gowns and aprons
- protective headwear
- masks
- protective eyewear
- protective footwear.

Medium risk category

Where exposure to high risk body fluids may occur but spattering is unlikely, gloves should be worn. Aprons, masks and protective eyewear should be available, for example, during the insertion or removal of intravascular devices (venous and arterial).

Low risk category

Where exposure to high risk body fluids is unlikely or is easily contained, gloves need not be worn but should be available, for example, intramuscular, intradermal or subcutaneous injections.

No risk category

Where there is no risk of exposure to 'high risk' body fluids, for example, taking an X-ray where no invasive procedure is performed. Normal hand-washing procedures are adequate.

All health care providers working with children and young people should know that protective clothing may seem very threatening to the child. Reassurance and explanations will be necessary to allay their fears.

Protective clothing

It is essential that protective clothing should be removed after the procedure or on leaving the contaminated area, in order to minimise the risk of spread of infection; for example, contaminated footwear can disseminate blood extensively. The use of disposable equipment such as gowns and drapes should be encouraged. Non-disposable protective wear such as eye protection, boots, etc., must be adequately cleaned and disinfected.

Gloves

The type of gloves used (surgical, examination or household) will depend on the task involved. A specification for non-sterile, natural rubber latex examination gloves has been published by the Department of Health[3].

Moulded latex gloves should be worn whenever a procedure involving sharp instruments is undertaken or where there is a likelihood of blood soiling. In the event of the user being unable to wear latex rubber because of allergic reactions, advice should be obtained from the Occupational Health Department. Plastic or vinyl gloves may be a suitable alternative. It is advisable that gloves should be worn in the following circumstances.

- For all procedures where contamination with blood is probable.
- During venepuncture. It is recognised that the veins of babies and infants are difficult to palpate and gloves may possibly hinder the procedure, therefore the risk factors should be assessed by the person performing the procedure and individual decisions made within the recommendations of the local policy on control of infection.
- For handling soiled dressings etc., if a 'non-touch' technique is not used.
- For handling excretions/secretions where any microbial contamination of the hands may occur.
- For cleaning of spillages of body fluid.
- For a child who has diarrhoea.
- For cleaning equipment prior to disinfection/sterilisation.
- For handling chemical disinfectants.

It must be emphasised that any body fluid may represent a potential source of both hospital and community acquired infection. Thus, handwashing is indicated following contact with these substances – even when using gloves. Gloves should be discarded between patients as it has been demonstrated that nosocomial (hospital acquired) pathogens can adhere to the glove even after washing[4].

Water-repellent gowns and aprons

There are many disposable waterproof or water-repellent gowns commercially available. Some have reinforced sleeves and front panels which are more comfortable to wear. They may be obtained in sterile and non-sterile form from the relevant manufacturers.

Disposable plastic aprons should be readily available and can be worn during any dirty procedures. Some paediatric nurses are concerned about the unpleasantness of cuddling a baby next to plastic, or of the risk of the baby slipping. There are disposable aprons which have a rougher surface and slipping is less likely, but these are more expensive. In the author's experience, slipping has not proved to be a problem.

Disposable gowns or aprons should be used in the following circumstances.

- For all procedures where contamination of blood is probable and spattering is likely to occur.
- During all dirty procedures, including cleaning equipment prior to disinfection or sterilisation.
- When handling chemicals where accidental spattering may occur.

Protective headwear

Where the risk of gross contamination with blood is likely, for example, in the operating theatre, appropriate gowns/suits with attachable hoods should be available. As an alternative, disposable hats may be worn.

Masks

Where the risk of splashing blood into the face or mucosal surfaces (eye, nose, mouth) exists, for example, during dental procedures or bronchoscopy, a disposable filter mask – commonly used in operating theatres – should be worn.

Protective eyewear

Protective spectacles, goggles or a visor should be worn where there is a risk of spattering of blood or chemicals into the eyes, for example, during some major surgical procedures or endoscopy examinations, especially bronchoscopy, delivering babies, and when handling gluteradehyde, etc. All equipment must be adequately cleaned and disinfected after use. If it is grossly contaminated then incineration should be considered. (Protective eyewear should be British Standard approved.)

Protective footwear

Theatre boots/shoes must be worn when contamination of blood is likely to occur, for example, when carrying out major surgical or obstetric procedures. The protective boots/shoes must be adequately cleaned and disinfected after use. Disposable overshoes provide less protection.

Avoiding exposure to sharps and needlestick injuries

Surveillance studies suggest that HIV is not easily transmitted in the health-care setting, but needlstick injuries predominate as a cause of occupationally acquired HIV infection. Figures suggest that following a needlestick injury with known HIV antibody-positive source there is a less than one in 200 chance of the injured person becoming infected by HIV, whereas in hepatitis B, carriers of this virus have a 20 per cent risk of infecting the health care worker who has sustained an inoculation injury[5].

Care should always be taken to avoid other means of exposure, for example, to mucous membranes, conjunctiva, broken skin with blood, or blood-stained body fluids, as cases of transmission through this route have been demonstrated.

All health care workers should be individually responsible for the safe disposal of sharps and must not put other staff at risk through carelessness and neglect. Needles must not be resheathed unless by a safe method with suitable equipment. Disposable needles, syringes and other disposable sharps such as scalpel blades, stitch cutters, etc., must be placed promptly in a puncture-resistant bin which is suitable for incineration. The British Standard for Sharps Containers is now available along with the DHSS specification for sharps containers (TSS/S/330.015) and should be noted[6]. These bins must *never* be overfilled. Dirty, used needles and other sharps protruding from overloaded sharps bins are dangerous and increase the risk of inoculation injury.

Inoculation injury

When sustaining an inoculation injury, splashing of blood into the mucosal surfaces or onto intact skin, immediate first aid action must be taken.

- For inoculation injury: allow the blood to flow freely. Do not suck the wound. Wash well with cold running tap water and soap.
- For mucous membrane exposure:
  — Splashes into the mouth – wash out with copious amounts of running tap water. Do not swallow.
  — Splashes into the eyes – irrigate with running tap water or eye-wash facilities using normal saline.
- Skin exposure: thoroughly wash the area with running tap water and soap.

Any incidents of this kind must be reported immediately to the management and Occupational Health Department and an incident form completed. The local employer's philosophy and policy should be referred to where necessary.

It should be emphasised that all health care providers working with patients and potentially infected body fluids should be strongly advised to have hepatitis B vaccination and should be followed up with their informed consent with regard to their antibody/immunity status.

It should be recognised by everyone concerned that considerable anxiety can be provoked by sharps injuries involving blood, especially when the source of blood is unknown or known to be HIV antibody-positive. This is not surprising and it is important that anxiety is allowed to be expressed.

When the incident occurs the doctor of the patient concerned should be consulted about risk factors. However, testing the patient for HIV may not provide an answer because of the 'window period' (see Chapter 2). This is the time between initial infection and sero-conversion, when antibodies will form. This period may last for approximately three months. Views vary about the exact length of time it takes for HIV antibodies to be detected after transmission. Young babies may test positive for HIV antibodies for a considerable period of time due to the presence of maternal antibodies; they may never develop their own antibodies and may in fact be HIV negative. It should be emphasised that if the HIV status of any patient is not known, the correct procedures, which include gaining informed and counselled parental consent to test for HIV, are of paramount importance. If this consent is not obtained and a child is tested for HIV, there may be dire consequences: parental positive HIV status may be discovered and the ensuing trauma and possible litigation could be a very real possibility.

After specific counselling, the health care worker can be offered baseline antibody testing which, if negative, can be repeated at 6 weeks, 12 weeks and 6 months, together with medical support and advice. If the health care worker remains HIV negative, they may be considered to be uninfected by the exposure. An alternative procedure would be to store a serum sample and it can be tested if the individual becomes unwell. Occupational exposure to HIV-infected blood should be reported to CDSC where details are recorded in strict confidence using a coded system[7].

The issue of whether zidovudine (AZT) should be given as prophylaxis to a person who has had an incident with a known HIV antibody-positive blood should be addressed[8]. It has been suggested that zidovudine could be beneficial in incidents of this kind. There has been no published evidence to support this form of treatment. The risks of using the drug have to be weighed against the possible benefits as there are acknowledged side effects. The safety of this drug has *not* been established in pregnancy.

Because of the complexity of the issues and the suggestion that the drug should be started quickly (within two hours) and continued for six weeks, it is important that no time is wasted. The person should be given the opportunity of receiving the drug if they so wish and if it is indicated. The Communicable Disease Surveillance Centre (CDSC) for England, Wales and Northern Ireland and Communicable Disease (Scotland) Unit, Glasgow will be prepared to give advice and there is usually a doctor on call. It is advisable for the health-care worker to obtain advice before making any informed decision.

Implementing an effective standard of hygiene

In order to reduce the risk of exposure and transmission of blood-borne pathogens and other micro-organisms, the general principles of good infection control practice must be followed. Attention is drawn to the following areas where concern has been expressed by health care workers.

Hand hygiene

Cuts or other skin lesions should be covered with a waterproof plaster. Health care workers suffering from exfoliate determatitis or similar skin conditions should be advised not to handle potentially infected material and further advice should be sought from the local Occupational Health Department. Regular handwashing should be undertaken before and after all clinical procedures and also after handling contaminated or dirty materials during such tasks. Protective gloves should be worn when handling infected or potentially infected material[9].

Disinfection and sterilisation methods

General principles

Manufacturers' instructions must be followed as there may be contra-indications to various methods of decontamination. All equipment should be well maintained[10]. Heat is the best method of disinfection and should always be used where it is practical[11,12]. All equipment must be washed in hot water and detergent, rinsed and dried *before* embarking on disinfection or sterilisation. Chemical disinfection should not be used unless there is no alternative method of decontamination. When using chemical disinfectants, check:

- that organic matter has been removed. Most disinfectants are inactivated by grease and dirt.
- the expiry date
- the correct dilution and immersion time
- the manufacturer's instructions
- that appropriate protective clothing is worn
- that care is taken with electrical equipment.

For the purposes of rendering an item safe for patient use, it needs to be:

- Clean (the physical removal of soil and organic material from items/objects), or
- Disinfected (the removal or destruction of harmful micro-organisms, but not bacterial spores), or
- Sterilised (the complete destruction or removal of all living micro-organisms including bacterial spores).

The process used depends on the risk of infection involved in the use of the item: this is therefore divided into three categories.

(i)   *High risk items.* These are items which directly or indirectly come into contact with either tissue and/or blood and body fluids, for example, surgical instruments, cardiac/urinary catheters, implants, needles, or other susceptible body sites, for example, traumatised tissue. High risk items must be sterilised.

(ii)   *Medium risk items.* These are items which directly or indirectly have contact with intact mucous membrane, for example, anaesthetic equipment, bronchoscopes, thermometers, as well as bedpans, potties etc. Medium risk items need not be sterile, but must be disinfected.

As children often put things in their mouths, it is accepted that objects such as toys need only be socially clean, unless contaminated with blood, other body fluid or faecal matter.

(iii)   *Low risk items.* These are items which touch only intact skin or make no contact with the patient, for example, blood pressure cuffs, furniture, etc. Low risk items must be kept clean and dry.

Heat is the best method of disinfection and should always be used where practical. HIV and hepatitis viruses, together with most other organisms affecting patients with AIDS, are susceptible to heat.

Boiling will inactivate both HIV and hepatitis B viruses, although it must be emphasised that bacterial spores may not be destroyed. The previously cleaned instrument should be totally immersed in the water and all air bubbles expelled. The temperature of the water must be 100°C for at least five minutes. A purpose-built electric instrument boiler may be used, or a modified commercial pressure-cooker with appropriate safety features can be used as an alternative for general practice, dental and family planning practice[13,14]. (Used instruments such as vaginal speculae can also be disinfected by this method.)

Although hepatitis B requires a higher temperature than HIV for inactivation, the action of the washing process together with the correct temperatures are deemed to be adequate. Most steam bedpan disinfectors reach a temperature of 80°C for one minute, and washing machines, including domestic machines can reach a temperature of 65°C for 10 minutes (Table 12.2).

Table 12.2   Recommended minimum temperatures for sterilisation

	Temperature (°C)	*Holding time (minutes)*
Moist heat	134	3
	126	10
	121	15
	115	30
Dry heat	180	30
	160	60
For disinfection:		
Boiling	100	5
Washing machines	80	1
	71	3
	65	10

Chemical disinfection should only be undertaken in the absence of any other suitable method. When using this method, the following additional points must be considered:

- the variable effects on different micro-organisms
- incompatibility with various materials
- reduced efficacy in the presence of organic matter
- susceptibility to deterioration with storage and dilution
- toxic potential.

The following disinfectants are advised for the inactivation of HIV and hepatitis viruses[15,16].

Hypochlorite

Fresh solutions of sodium hypochlorite or sodium dichloroisocyanurate tablets or granules are recommended for general surface disinfection. The dilution of the chemical is shown in Table 12.3 below.

It is recommended that surfaces likely to become contaminated should be covered with a disposable impermeable covering or a tray which can be sterilised. The surface underneath should be wiped over with a 0.1 per cent (1000 ppm) solution using a disposable cloth. Non-autoclavable equipment, e.g. stethoscopes, may be decontaminated using a 0.1% solution with a minimum contact time of 30 minutes.

Blood spillages

Spillages of blood should be dealt with as soon as possible. The contaminated area should be completely covered with a 1% hypochlorite solution (10000 ppm) or granules/powder of a similar concentration. The area should be wiped up with a gloved hand using disposable paper towels which are then discarded into a clinical waste bag. The area should then be washed with hot water and detergent, and dried in order to reduce the risk of surface damage. Hypochlorite has the disadvantage of being corrosive to metal, bleaching to fabrics and damaging to rubber.

Table 12.3 Dilution of hypochlorite solutions for decontamination

	Per cent dilution	Parts per million of available chlorine
Blood spillage	1	10000
Potentially contaminated surfaces	0.1	1000

Gluteraldehyde

A two per cent solution is currently recommended for fibre-optic endoscopes[17]. All channels should be cleaned and disinfected and a fully immersible endoscope and an automatic cleaning machine should be used wherever possible. Non-immersible endoscopes must be cleaned and disinfected manually by a similar process.

After use on a known case of mycobacterial infection (tuberculosis) or *Cryptosporidia* infection, the time of gluteraldehyde exposure of endoscopes should be increased to 60 minutes[18,19]. Endoscopes which will enter sterile body cavities must normally be immersed for a minimum of three hours (see Table 12.4).

Alcohol

This is not recommended for disinfecting the surfaces of equipment or work

Table 12.4 Recommended sterilisation procedures

Equipment	Comments
Flexible fibre-optic gastrointestinal endoscopes	The Working Party of the British Society for Gastroenterology 1988 recommends a short period of exposure to disinfection (four minutes) as a routine between patients, provided the instrument is well cleaned before disinfection. A longer period of exposure (10 minutes) may be preferred at the beginning and end of a list, to eleminate bacteria that may multiply in the stored instrument and present a risk to immuno-suppressed patients
Cystoscopes	Immersion time 10 minutes minimum
Bronchoscopes	Immersion time 20–30 minutes

benches contaminated with blood. It should only be used on equipment which is incompatible with the above disinfectants. Seventy per cent ethanol can be used to irrigate channels in some fibre-optic endoscopes and it must remain in contact with the surfaces for at least two minutes. The cleaning of the insertion tube and wiping of the surface with 70 per cent ethanol will remove most micro-organisms, but its use against HIV if doubtful. Other items may be immersed in 70 per cent Isopropanol or Industrial Methylated Spirits for a minimum of one hour.

Maintaining an effective standard of hygiene

Disposal of clinical waste

All waste which is contaminated with blood must be considered potentially infected and treated as 'clinical waste' in accordance with the Health Services Advisory Committee's document 'The safe disposal of clinical waste'[20,21]. It is important that sharps, blood-stained material or other infected waste are safely contained until they can be incinerated.

Decontamination of laundry

All infected and blood-stained laundry should be processed as directed in the document 'Hospital laundry arrangements for used and infected linen'[21]. All blood-stained and infected laundry should be safely contained in the appropriate coloured bag until it is effectively washed. Linen may be decontaminated in a washing machine that reaches temperatures of at least 65°C for 10 minutes or 71°C for 3 minutes. Although hepatitis B virus requires a higher temperature, the action of the washing process at these temperatures is felt to be adequate.

In the community, linen and bedding that is blood-stained should be washed in a well maintained machine, rinsing initially in the cold rinse cycle and then in the hot wash cycle (approximately 80°C). Overloading of the machine must be avoided. If washing by hand is unavoidable, household rubber gloves must be worn. The hot water and detergent should be as hot as can be tolerated and the linen rinsed in hot water.

Crockery, cutlery and other feeding equipment

This should be washed in a dishwasher. Where this is not possible, wash in hot water and detergent, rinse in separate hot water and then dry. Disposable utensils are not necessary. Babies feeding equipment should be cleaned and sterilised, where appropriate, in the usual way.

Bedpans, urinals, vomit bowls, etc.

This equipment should be disinfected by the routine hospital system in an efficient washer-disinfector that achieves temperatures of 80°C for one minute. Excrement can be put into the normal sewage system via the toilet or sluice.

Disposable equipment may be discarded in a macerator in the normal manner. The bedpan holder must be washed in hot water and detergent and dried after use. Care should be taken to avoid splashing when disposing of excreta.

The bowl of a commode should be washed in a hot wash machine as above. Where this is not possible, it should be washed with gloved hands in hot water and detergent, rinsed and dried. The surface of the commode should be cleaned with hypochlorite-based sanitiser, rinsed and wiped dry. Equipment used at home may be cleaned as above.

Added specific precautions in specialised areas of work

Operating theatre

The consultant in charge of the patient should be responsible for seeing that all members of the team know of the risk of infection and of measures to be taken. The team should be limited to essential members of staff only, if there is a child at risk with HIV infection due to undergo surgical procedures. It should be mentioned that patients whose HIV status is unknown and who undergo surgery, may care to prevent cross-infection should be taken at all times for all patients.

Pre-operative shaving should be avoided where possible and a depilatory cream used where hair removal is essential.

It is not essential for children known to have HIV to be placed at the end of an operating list, providing adequate cleaning and decontamination of equipment is performed between cases.

- Unnecessary equipment should be removed and disposable drapes and equipment used where possible.
- The mattress on the operating table should be protected with an impermeable disposable sheeting.
- Appropriate protective clothing must be worn by members of the team. The surgeons may wish to use double gloves as this may minimise the risk of inoculation injury.

A measured quantity of sodium hypoclorite solution should be put into the suction bottles to increase the inactivation of the virus. After use, the contents of these jars must be carefully emptied down the sluice hopper, taking care to avoid personal and environmental contamination. Protective clothing must be worn. Variations in operative technique which reduce the risk of inoculation are:

- a non-touch approach
- the avoidance of passing sharp instruments from surgeon to nurse and vice versa
- new techniques in cutting (as with lasers) or of wound closure that obviate the use of sharp instruments.

Staff should be experienced in the handling of surgical instruments/tools. Unwashed instruments etc., should be contained in a robust leak-proof container and prior to sterilisation/disinfection either:

- sent to the hospital or theatre Sterile Services Unit in a sealed container for decontamination. The container may be labelled 'danger of infection'. However, it must be emphasised that *all* blood-stained equipment must be handled in a safe manner. The practice of immersing dirty instruments in a chemical disinfectant prior to cleaning is felt to be unnecessary;
- placed in a washing machine prior to sterilisation/disinfection;
- washed by hand, taking care to avoid inoculation injury and splashing.

Closed rather than open wound drainage is recommended. Blood should be cleaned off the patient's skin at the end of the operation. A wound dressing should be used which will contain exudate with an outer impermeable cover.

Maternity units and family planning clinics

Protective clothing should be worn by all staff performing vaginal examinations and attending the delivery. Care must also be taken when handling the placenta and lochia. The placenta should be wrapped in an impermeable plastic bag and incinerated. (See also Chapter 6.)

Sanitary towels should be placed in a plastic bag and incinerated. For further information see the document *HIV Infection in Maternity Care and Gynaecology: a Report of the RCOG Sub-committee on Problems Associated with AIDS in Relation to Obstetric and Gynaecology* (1990).

All clinical departments, including the Psychiatric Service

The measures to be taken by staff should be the same in all units:

- care with blood and sharps
- avoidance of injuries
- gloves for blood exposure
- covering cuts and open lesions.

Where invasive procedures are likely to be performed on an unco-operative person, for example, during venepuncture, the risk of accidental inoculation injury may be decreased by the availability of sufficient staff.

Accommodation in hospital for children with HIV

In most circumstances, no special precautions need be taken other than those for handling blood and body fluids. The following categories of isolation are recommended[22].

(i)   Children who are HIV antibody positive and who may or may not have generalised persistent lymphadenopathy without immune suppression, need only be nursed in single rooms in the following circumstances:

- if bleeding occurs or is likely to occur
- if diarrhoea is present

- following surgery, if external bleeding is likely to occur
- for any child requiring privacy for specific reasons.

The child should be allowed to mix with other children when they have recovered from the above conditions, unless the child has diarrhoea due to an infective agent such as salmonella. Young children in nappies or who are incontinent are more likely to spread pathogens from person to person than an older child who understands the principles of hygiene and handwashing after going to the toilet.

They may be allowed to participate in normal and social activities on the ward such as playing, eating, bathing and toileting.

(ii)   Those children who present with the clinical syndrome of AIDS or AIDS-related complex should preferably be nursed in a single room. The child may be infected with opportunistic infections such as salmonella or tuberculosis with the increased risk of infecting a susceptible population on the ward. Likewise, common childhood illnesses such as chickenpox, measles and viral diarrhoea are commonplace in a paediatric ward and morbidity and mortality of the immuno-suppressed child is increased with these infections.

Accommodation for parents should be made available in order for them to continue to nurse the child if they so wish. Consideration should be given to the parents, who may be infected themselves, in providing facilities so that they can continue to minimise the risk of infection in their normal daily routine; for example, facilities for disposing of sanitary towels, or for the continuing use of their own intravenous drug therapy. There should be provision made for any other ongoing maintenance treatment they require, where appropriate.

Community care

Many children with HIV/AIDS and other communicable infectious agents are nursed safely in their homes. The same principles of infection control measures can be applied in the home setting without restricting normal social activities. There is no evidence that social contact with others presents a risk of transmission of HIV infection.

Normal domestic methods of hygiene and waste disposal will suffice with people who are asymptomatic. Advice should be given with regard to not sharing items such as razors or toothbrushes. Women should dispose of used sanitary towels/tampons either by burning or by flushing down the toilet.

For those children and/or adults who have AIDS or HIV-related illnesses and require nursing at home, it may be necessary for arrangements to be made with the local authority for the collection of waste for incineration and for the laundering of infected linen. It is important that the rules of confidentiality should not be broken and any information given to external agencies may need to be discussed and clarified with the child's family before a relevant referral is made. In some instances, yellow bags have been left outside the house for collection, and the home has become a target for victimisation. This situation may be remedied with anticipation and careful negotiation and planning. Community staff should ensure they have sufficient and appropriate protective clothing and facilities for disinfection where needed (household bleach diluted 1 : 10 with water will suffice)[23]. Incineration of 'sharps bins' can be arranged at the nearest health clinic or hospital.

Any non-disposable or non-autoclavable nursing equipment which has been used must be decontaminated before re-use in accordance with local infection control policies. Further advice may be sought from the Senior Nurse, Infection Control, or the Infection Control Officer.

Transportation of specimens

Advice is given in the Health Services Advisory Committee document *Safety in Health Service Laboratories: the Labelling, Transport and Reception of specimens*, 1986, HMSO. Specimens must be in screw-capped, leak-proof containers and placed in individual sealed plastic bags. The accompanying laboratory form must be kept separate from the specimen in the plastic bag and both should be labelled with a bio-hazard warning label.

Specimens to be sent by post should be packed as described in current Post Office regulations.

Death of a child with regard to control of infection

Relatives and friends who wish to pay their last respects to the child should be allowed to do so in the normal way. Parents, siblings and significant others known well to the child may require a quiet and private time with the child after death has occurred. It is preferable to allow them to be with the child at the bedside. It may have been possible to explain previously that, due to HIV infection, there may be certain restrictions about embalming and viewing the body after it has left the ward. In some circumstances, it is possible for funeral directors to facilitate a further opportunity for the family to see the child's body. Staff or relatives who carry out last offices should wear protective clothing. Unless the death has been reported to the coroner, all drains and catheters etc., should be removed and disposed of as clinical waste. Leaking wounds must be closed with a waterproof dressing. Care must be taken to minimise the leakage of any body fluid. As in life, care should be taken to avoid contamination with blood and other body fluids[24].

The body should be laid out according to local policy taking into account the cultural and spiritual needs of the family. The embalming of known or suspected HIV-infected bodies is not recommended, but if essential for cultural reasons, particular attention must be given to avoid contamination and the work must be performed by experienced staff.

The body is then placed in a plastic cadaver bag and both the body and the bag labelled 'danger of infection'. These are obtainable specifically for babies and children. If there is a need for relatives to view the body at a later stage, then respect for their feelings must be observed and the bag opened appropriately. Good communication regarding the risks of infection must be maintained with mortuary staff and others who may be handling the body.

Many people understandably react emotionally towards this practice. It should be performed with the utmost sensitivity and respect for the child, the family and the health care worker.

Training programmes for all health care workers

The key to the control of any infectious disease is understanding how it is spread. Health care workers have different jobs, different training needs and different standards of practice. However, it is not acceptable for different people to practice different methods of control. This only helps to create confusion and fear, and leads to diminishing credibility in the eyes of the public.

The only method of controlling disease is through education. The principles of infection control should be taught to parents and children as well as to all health care providers. Where possible, the practices should be the same at home as in hospital. Where they are different, a full explanation must be given to the family in order that they fully understand the reasons for any necessary precautions.

Information about HIV should be targeted at children and adolescents in order that their attitudes towards infection control and 'safe sex' are not coloured by myth and fear. (See Chapter 8, Part 2).

Health authorities have a responsibility to ensure that all employees are adequately trained for the job they are employed to do. This means that all unit managers are responsible for ensuring their staff are given the opportunity, and positively encouraged, to attend training programmes. Working methods, procedures and policies should be updated regularly and be readily available for staff to read.

The main challenge to those concerned with control of infection is to ensure that what we already know is implemented effectively. It is not just a matter of scientific knowledge, but a matter of political and personal will.

References

1. Centers for Disease Control Update (1988). Universal precautions for prevention of transmission of human immunodeficiency virus, hepatitis B virus and other blood borne pathogens in health care settings. *Morbidity and Mortality Weekly Report*, **37**, 377–88.
2. Expert Advisory Group on AIDS (1990). *Guidance for Clinical Health Care Workers. Protection Against Infection with HIV and Hepatitis Viruses*, HMSO, London.
3. DOH Specification TSS/D/300.010 (1988). *NHS Procurement Directorate Specification for Non-sterile Natural Rubber Latex Examination Gloves*, HMSO, London.
4. Doebbeling, B.N., Pfaller, M.A., Houston, A.K., Wenzel, R.P. (1988). Removal of nosocomial pathogens from the contaminated glove: implications for glove re-use and handwashing. *Annals of International Medicine*, **109**, 394–8.
5. Gerberding, J.L., Bryant-Le Blanc, C.E., Nelson, K. *et al.* (1987). Risk of transmitting the human immunodeficiency virus, cytomegalovirus and hepatitis B virus to health-care workers exposed to patients with AIDS and AIDS-related conditions. *Journal of Infectious Diseases*, **156**, 1–8.
6. DHSS Specification No. TSS/S/300.015 (1982). *Specification for Containers for the Disporal of Used Needles and Sharp Instruments*.
7. Marcus, R. and the CDC (1988). Co-operative needlestick surveillance group. Surveillance of health care workers exposed to blood from patients infected with the human immunodeficiency virus. *New England Journal of Medicine*, **319**, 1118–23.
8. Henderson, D.K. and Gerberding, J.L. (1989). Prophylactic zidovudine after occupational exposure to the human immunodeficiency virus: An interim analysis. *Journal of Infectious Diseases*, **160(2)**, 321–7.
9. Taylor, L. (1978). An evaluation of handwashing techniques. *Nursing Times*, **74(2)**, 54–5 and **(3)**, 108–9.
10. DHSS NH (87) 22 (1987). *Decontamination of Health Care Equipment Prior to Inspection, Service or Repair*, HMSO, London.
11. Aycliffe, G.A.J., Coates, D., Hoffman, P.N. (1984). *Public Health Laboratory. Chemical Disinfection in Hospitals*.
12. Hoffman, P.N. (1988). Control of infection in general practice: a survey and recommendation. *British Medical Journal*, **297**, 34–6.

13. *A Code of Practice for Sterilisation of Instruments and Control of Cross Infection* (June 1989): BMA, London.
14. DHSS Health Equipment Information No. 185 (1988). *An Evaluation of Portable Steam Sterilisers for Unwrapped Instruments and Utensils*, HMSO, London.
15. Hanson, P.J.V., Gor, D., Jeffries, D.J. (1989). Chemical inactivation of HIV on surfaces. *British Medical Journal*, **298**, 862–4.
16. DOH Health Notice HN (87) 1 (1987). *Decontamination of Equipment Linen or Other Surfaces Contaminated with Hepatitis B or HIV*, DOH, London.
17. Working Party of British Society for Gastroenterology (1988). Cleaning and disinfection of equipment for gastrointestinal flexible endoscopy – interim recommendations. *Gut*, **29**, 1134–51.
18. DOH Safety Information SIB (86) 34 (May 1986). *Disinfection of Endoscopes Potentially Contaminated with Mycobacterium Species*, DOH, London.
19. Research Committee of British Thoracic Society Working Party (1988). Broncoscopy and infection control. *Lancet*, 270–1.
20. DHSS HN (82) 22 (1982). *Disposal of Clinical Waste*, HMSO, London.
21. DHSS HC (FP) 87/5 (1987). *Disposal of Clinical Waste from General Medicine and General Dental Practice Premises*, HMSO, London.
22. Macqueen, S. (1989). Positive practice. *Nursing Times*, **85(43)**, 67–8.
23. Coates, D. (1988). Household bleaches and HIV. *Journal of Hospital Infection*, **11**, 95–7.
24. DOH (1978). *Code of Practice for the Prevention of Infection in Clinical Laboratories and Post Mortem Rooms*, HMSO, London.

Further reading

A Guide to the Health and Safety (Dangerous Pathogens) Regulations (1981). Health and Safety Executive (H and S. booklet Hs (R) 12 1981).
Caddow, P. (1989). *Applied Microbiology*, Scutari Press, London.
Andre Brenda Ciak (1988). AIDS attitudes and infection control. *American Journal of Infection Control*, **16(6)**, 272–3.
Control of Substances Hazardous to Health Regulations (1988). Statutory Instrument No. 1657.
Gee, G., Moran, T.A. (1988). *AIDS – Concepts in Nursing Practice*, Williams and Wilkins, USA.
Hudson, C.N., Sharp, F. (1988). *AIDS and Obstetric and Gynaecology*, Royal College of Obstetricians and Gynaecologists, London.
Pratt, R.J. (1991). *AIDS: A Strategy for Nursing Care*, 3rd Edn, Edward Arnold, Sevenoaks.
Technical Panel on Infections within Hospitals – American Hospital Association (1989). Management of HIV infection in the hospital. *American Journal of Infection Control*, **17(4)**, 24A–44A.

The thoughts and feelings of families affected by HIV disease

The following contributions have been written by people whose families are affected by HIV infection and AIDS. This writing was difficult and painful, but the authors offered their contributions in the hope that the knowledge of their own experiences might give others some insight into the lives of families living with HIV disease.

The need for confidentiality has been respected. The names of family members have been changed to protect their identity.

Ed.

This is the transcript of a tape sent to one of the editors of this book by a friend – he is the father of Tommy who has haemophilia and HIV.

I think the first thing I would like to do is make an apology for taking so long to get this together. It was no deliberate act. It was just something I found very difficult to do – but yes, I wanted to do it.

Okay – enough of this banter. Let's try and get on with this thing I'm trying to avoid. I'll just say it as it comes into my head. I will refer to myself as Keith, and I will refer to my son as Tommy. I'll explain that later if I may.

Oh Lord – where do I start? We're a family. There's my wife, myself and our three children. The eldest is a girl, not long turned sixteen, the next in line is a boy who'll be thirteen this year, and then there's the youngest who was nine three days ago. The next year or two will be a part of my life I will regret for as long as I live – because that is the expected time that we have left as a family – my wife, myself and our three children.

Tommy was born nine years ago, tested for haemophilia and found to be affected. The reason for the test was that my wife is a proven carrier of haemophilia and her father died of the disease. He was found to be 5% which is not terribly severe. I think they consider it moderately acute, but that's all.

Tommy's childhood accident record is one that we are rather proud of. On only four occasions up to the age of four and a half years of age, he needed just four injections of Factor VIII. The record would show that they were typical childhood ailments – learning to crawl, bumping into furniture, banging his head – that kind of situation.

In fact, when he was four and a half the injection that infected him with HIV was for a bitten tongue. Silly, isn't it. We just couldn't stop the tongue from bleeding (due to his haemophilia) and we took him to the hospital and, as parents, you feel you make all the right moves. They gave him the injection. Shortly after that he was given a test for HIV without our knowledge and found to be positive. We were informed of this by a letter. I still have that letter.

Not long after that, the hospital felt they should gather the parents into groups and hold a meeting, and basically the doctor at the time explained that 'although we feel it will make absolutely no difference in any way, shape or form to your children, we feel we are obliged to legally inform you that something has been introduced into their blood stream which wasn't there before. It was a pure accident, but it should make absolutely no difference to the child, whatsoever. Does anybody have any questions?'

Well, that was probably a very easy time for the hospital because nobody had any knowledge of HIV then. I mean, ignorance was bliss. You didn't know what to ask.

At about five and a half years of age Tommy started to have constant ailments. Typical childhood problems – ear infections, chest infections, a variety of things, but they were permanent. He required treatment all the time and his condition deteriorated to the point where on March 18th 1988, the senior doctor explained to my wife and myself that Tommy now has AIDS related complex or ARC.

I won't say we were totally ignorant of the facts, but that was a shock. We really didn't suspect. It sounds silly, but we felt we were just having a bad time with a little boy who had lots of problems. It sounds a bit negative doesn't it, but anyway that was in 1988.

From there on, I think it's fair to say that he's deteriorated. It's affected his liver, his spleen, his kidneys – he's stopped growing and he's losing weight constantly. It's gradual, it's slow but it's constant – he's more or less permanently unwell.

There are times when he's forced to use a wheelchair. One particular morning comes to mind. It was painful to watch. He has problems with his glands – they swell in his groin and places like that and it's really painful for him to use his legs and put weight on them. This particular morning he'd woken up and decided he wanted to watch cartoons on the television in the lounge. Because he couldn't walk, he lay on the floor and pulled himself along by his arms. That was quite a major thing, and it brings a reality to a situation. You start to see things that aren't visually apparent. You're told things, you're attentive, but as a lay man, the words don't have the impact or effect that medical knowledge would give them. So you are interested, you do listen and you say yes when you feel you should, but you honestly don't totally understand. If you ask someone to explain things, they do, but you still haven't really understood.

The major heartbreak we had was when the hospital advised us to inform our other children of his terminal condition, as the hospital felt that Tommy's brother and sister were entitled to prepare themselves for what would shortly become visually apparent. That's what I mean. We don't fully understand. We know things are going to happen, we know it won't be nice, but we're not sure what to expect.

However, we debated at some length whether to tell our other children but felt the doctors, as professionals, would be right in their judgement. We felt the best way to do this would be to tell them separately. So one night when both the boys had gone to bed, we sat with our daughter and turned the television off and we made a cup of tea, explaining that we wanted to have a talk. We told her what had happened calmly, frankly and honestly. We didn't point any verbal fingers in anger and play politics with it, or get into that side, we simply explained what had happened, and it was likely that her little brother would die within the next year or two. She didn't ask any questions, she just sat and listened, and during the course of the conversation her eyes filled with tears and they fell down her cheeks. She was silent after we'd finished. A short time went by, it felt like a long time, and she simply said

'Have you finished?' We said 'Yes'. She got up and walked out of the room. She was very, very deeply hurt and very upset. During the course of the conversation we did say to her that we also intended to tell our younger son, but because he was younger than her, we would have to pick the time and place. We weren't sure when that would be, so we didn't want her to discuss it with her elder brother, because it was quite possible that she would bring up the subject that he would now nothing at all about.

When the time came to tell our younger son (he was eleven) we went for a drive in the car. It's something we often enjoy doing together. I picked a quiet road, that way I could concentrate on what I said rather than my driving. I didn't look at him. I kept my eyes on the road and once again I explained, coolly, calmly and honestly that Tommy had something introduced into his blood by mistake and this was having a bad effect, and he would not live as long as we would hope. He was probably going to live with us for another year, or probably two. Towards the end of the conversation I looked over at him and what I saw made me stop the car straight away. This little eleven-year-old boy sat there. He was absolutely sobbing. His face will haunt me for the rest of my life. It was awash with pain, horrible horrible pain. I'd crucified him. I tried to get close, to cuddle, to comfort him, just to hold him and he screamed at me and said 'Why did you tell me?' He didn't want to know. He had no idea. He'd never suspected. Childhood logic, I suppose. He accepted the fact that some people needed a lot of treatment and some people don't. His brother needed a lot of treatment – he doesn't. What's the problem? It ripped him in half. He didn't eat, didn't sleep, he wouldn't play, he wouldn't sit with his brother, he wouldn't sit in the same room – he was scared, he was frightened.

He's come to terms with it now. They both have. There are benefits. Tommy is no angel. Frankly, I think he gets fed up with life at times. The other two are both a lot more tolerant now. It's easier for children. They don't have the memories or the imagination to think as adults do. They get upset at the thought of the loss of a member of their family. They don't visualise, as parents do, the pain, the funeral, the suffering, the death, the heartbreak.

My wife and myself attended a funeral for another little boy that we knew, and in conversation afterwards we both admitted to each other that it had felt like a rehearsal for what we are going to have to go through. I wept that day. God, I broke my heart. I didn't see the little boy's name on the coffin, I saw Tommy's name.

When I look at Tommy, I hurt. When he looks at me, I smile.

I recall talking to a group of people on one particular occasion. I tried to put the situation to them in a way that I felt that I understand. I said it was somewhat similar to a game of football. The main difference being, of course, that if I didn't like the game of football I could pick up the ball and walk off the pitch. I'd simply say I don't wish to play this game anymore. But the game that I play now has two sides, and the other team is life. My team is me. I have nobody else on my side, there are no reserves. When life fouls you and you go down, you have to pick yourself up. It's somewhat unfair because I can't win this game, I can only lose. I don't score goals. I don't gain points. There's no light at the end of this tunnel. The end of the tunnel is when the light goes out.

Of course, as any parents in our own particular position will tell you, they will carry on. They have to. There are other children in the family and you have a responsibility as a parent to the rest of your family. It's difficult times like right now, when you're alone. Everybody must have their own way of trying to cope.

I said at the beginning that there was a reason why I refer to my son as Tommy and myself as Keith – and Rosie, I know you won't print my name is . . . and his name is . . . That's on sunny days. But there's a dark side you see. Because of our particular situation, we have been approached on a number of occasions by the Press and we've co-operated anonymously. Unfortunately, the media want the bare facts, that's what makes stories. The person that talks to them is Keith, about little Tommy. You see I couldn't bare to read '. . .' and his son '. . .'. I think I can cope when I read about some guy called Keith and his little boy Tommy. It probably sounds silly, but it helps me. The psychiatrists would probably have another opinion about that. But, well, there you go.

I can only discuss how a carer might feel. I can't speak for Tommy. Obviously he suffers, but I can't discuss that. I don't suffer that way, I don't suffer physically. All my suffering is mental. I believe every parent in the land who has a sick child, picks that child up at times and thinks 'I wish it could be me'. 'Why can't I do it for them?' I've done that to him. Once again, it didn't score a goal. It was a nice thought. Didn't work the second time either. It doesn't mean you don't try anymore, but you start to lose hope, and with the hope goes the will, and what else is there in life.

As man and wife it puts us under pressure because of the stigma that surrounds AIDS. It's a very anti-social, unacceptable disease, and it scares the hell out of people. They are genuinely frightened that their children might catch something from somebody else's child, I understand their fear. People who do not understand about HIV and AIDS are genuinely frightened and concerned. I don't hold that against them.

To get back to my wife and myself. I believe that all people need to express themselves, but we never really can. We do not actually sit and discuss it between us. We can't. We've never discussed the fact that we can't, we just both accept the fact that we can't. It didn't need to be said. But wouldn't it be nice if, when we are out with friends, we could. It's a very common question unfortunately. The minute you meet a couple and you have a drink or something they say 'How's the family?' 'How are the kids?' You live a lie because Tommy's condition is fairly visual because of the wheelchair. People who know us used to genuinely ask 'What's wrong?' We've come up with yet another lie. We tell them that he's got leukaemia. That's acceptable, that is OK. Shame – but no problem. We still have neighbours. We don't have graffiti, poison-pen letters or obscene phone calls. That's not imagination talking, that's fact. It did happen to people I knew.

Yes, there's an awful lot of pressure. To be fair, all the staff at the hospital are very very kind and they always have time for us. The atmosphere is as good as can be generated under the circumstances. It would be silly to say Tommy looks forward to going to hospital. I don't think any child or any adult would relish injections, transfusions, blood tests, brain scans, psychology tests, psychiatrists, all the things he goes through, but he feels he has a lot of friends down at the hospital. I feel we've developed the situation as well as it could be, and that's a help. For although Tommy has never asked what's wrong with him, he's obviously aware that he requires a lot of treatment. We've always said to him 'You have bad blood'. He's grown up with that, he's accepted that, he doesn't question it. We don't volunteer any other answers. His brother and sister say the same. 'It's your blood, that's all'.

We have entered into trials and studies for no particular reason, we just decided that the cause was good. We were approached by the hospital and explained that yes, Tommy was terminally ill and they can't do anything for him, but fortunately children in his particular circumstances are rather few and far between. What they lack is background information which will help them with future cases. So we've offered to attend brain scans a couple of times a year, so that they can measure the deterioration in his brain. We also go to psychology tests, so they can measure the effect on this central nervous system. That's for the same reason. They can't help Tommy but the information they gather might well help other children in the future. No goals again I'm afraid. No points scored there either, but keep trying. You must.

I would like to back track on something I said earlier when I was discussing the fact that we'd informed our other children about Tommy's condition. I can't really convey with words what a horrible experience it was. Other parents may find themselves approaching a similar position. I would like to offer some advice or some help but I'm sorry I can't. There is none. I believe it's up to the individual family. We chose to tell Tommy's brother and sister for one main reason, which for me sways the argument more than any other point as to whether or not they should be informed. I believe that they are old enough to understand the situation. I believe they should know because when Tommy dies, if they found out that we knew he was going to die but didn't tell them, I feel they would be entitled to resent us, and for that one reason alone I believe they should know. That's our reason. It worked for us although it may not work for anybody else, and I wouldn't advise it for everyone.

As for the future it's a blank. No plans, no thoughts, simply don't think about it. Take one day at a time. We tend to split up our year. We look forward to the next birthday, the next holiday, Christmas, Easter. Each day or date we achieve is another milestone.

To be fair, all things considered, as a family we are extremely happy. This might sound a total contradiction allowing for what I have just said. What I've just said is the reality of the situation. It does not deny us the opportunity to function and be happy as a family, and we value and cherish our time. We make good use of it. We laugh a lot.

We've now come to terms with the fact that we're going to lose him. I accept it. I keep pausing the tape because while I'm discussing it I'm still crying about it. It still hurts as much today as the first day we were told 'He's terminal'. But I accept it.

There's nothing anybody, anywhere can do – the doctors can't, they want to, but they can't. I don't pursue religion, if it helps, do it. It wouldn't help me. People are kind, the nurses, the doctors, they do care. Most of them do understand, they will always listen, they will often give advice, they will help as much as anybody can.

When you go to bed at night, and you lie there in the dark, and the window of your mind starts rolling the pictures, your imagination steps in and you see what you see and you feel what you feel. Nobody can help. You're on you're own. Welcome to the game of football.

We are not unique as parents of children with AIDS. I just feel cheated because he wasn't born with a terminal condition. He was born quite normal and healthy. There was nothing to suspect he wouldn't live a normal healthy life. That's been taken away. I feel robbed . . .

The following contribution was written by Susie's mother.
Susie joined our family in 1987. She was nearly two years old, bright, plump and red-cheeked. She was also HIV positive.

Six months previously the Social Work Department had advertised a child in their regular Homefinder column in the local paper, and when I read about the baby who carried two viruses in her blood I was intrigued. I also knew what the viruses would be. My husband and I wanted another child to complete our family so we discussed the advertisement at length and responded hesitantly. The next six months seemed a lifetime as our application was processed and our suitability assessed. In an attempt to maintain our objectivity we were not allowed to meet Susie during this time, nor could we see photographs. The plan didn't work, she became very important to us very quickly.

The assessment period seemed agonisingly long and frustrating when we just wanted to bring Susie home, but with hindsight it was right. We were forced to examine our motives alone and together with professionals, to question our deepest beliefs on sensitive and serious issues like sickness and death, blame, guilt, responsibility and the basic rights of all people. We used the waiting time to learn, to gather information, contacts and telephone numbers. This time became a solid foundation of belief on which we were to base all our future decisions secure in the knowledge that we knew where we stood and how we got there.

Adapting to Susie was easy – no different to the arrival of any small child. Any adjustment in our lifestyle was for that reason only. Simple precautions became second nature, plastic gloves a routine item on the shopping list. Our son James, aged ten, easily accepted that Susie was to be treated with caution when she fell. For 18 months we were quietly happy with our circle of family and close friends. Susie was baptised, had birthday parties and family holidays. Concern about her health was manageable. Eventually though, it was time to enrol her in the local playgroup.

After taking advice from various experts and much discussion and heart-searching during our period of preparation we had reached the conclusion that Susie had the same right to medical confidentiality as everyone else. More importantly we had no right whatsoever, even as her parents, to breach that. After all, medical confidentiality is a basic tenet of our society and the means to protect other children were easy to understand, straightforward to administer and inexpensive. The necessary procedures had been extensively publicised through the media and by government AIDS education campaigns. Why then did we feel decidedly uneasy about approaching the playgroup? Because we suspected that it wasn't going to be that simple and our initial contact with the playgroup confirmed our suspicions. The group was completely unprepared and shocked that this could touch their lives.

Susie lost her privacy through ignorance and lack of forethought and we had our first, painful experience of society's assumption that, in the case of HIV infection as the exception among most other diseases, it had the right to know.

'Never mind' we said. 'When she enters the education system it will be different. The Education Authority is run by professionals, it is a statutory body and must surely be complying with the guidelines issued by the Scottish Office, among others?' And besides, three years ago the colleagues of these same professionals were assuring us that, in their opinion, our daughter was entitled to her privacy. Wrong again! Or rather, right – since we had already experienced the same feelings of unease which we recognised from before.

Good, clear, responsible guidelines existed but they weren't being implemented routinely! For the second time we faced the attitude that action would be taken when necessary, with the implication that *necessary* was when a child known to be HIV positive joined the school. Again we learned that both professional and lay people believed they would be told, should be told and had a right to be told. We also learned how frightened the professionals were of being 'blamed' if it came out that an HIV-positive child was within the group or school without the knowledge (and, I suspect, consent) of the staff and parents. There were occasional and heartwarming exceptions to this – people who were prepared to acknowledge Susie's rights and shoulder the responsibility in the face of any subsequent criticism, but they were very much the minority.

The focus was and, to a certain extent, still is on the child they know to be HIV positive and not on the risk from the ones they don't know about, even when asked what steps they intend to take to protect themselves and the children from the risk of an undiagnosed child or adult being within the group or school. It seems this scenario is beyond their imagination.

We speak out now. We've nothing to lose and maybe, by doing so, we can prevent another family from being exposed to public scrutiny with all the risks this entails. Susie has her label now and most people accept it kindly. How ungrateful we must seem when our thanks for their kindness and their interest is tinged with resentment that they have this information about our daughter in the first place. Don't they ask her to parties, invite her to play and generally treat her in the same way as they treat other children? Why then do we smile weakly when asked how others treat us and Susie? We reply that they are very kind and all the while we rage inside because we have to be grateful, because we shouldn't need the kindness which demands comment, because they had no right to know in the first place and their kindness is only good when compared to how life would be if they had been hostile. Don't they understand that by demanding the right to choose to be kind or otherwise they took away her right to privacy and unquestioned acceptance – her normality? Susie's normal life is now a gift given by others, one they can withdraw. It isn't hers by right. Will she one day need to feel grateful for acceptance? Real acceptance will only come when people can say 'I don't need to know who or where. I just need to be sure that throughout the system, my children are protected against the possibility of cross infection.' Until then, society cannot be trusted to behave well and although, with information about a particular person, most people will make an effort to overcome their natural early fears, some won't. We know how difficult this can be, this waiting to see if you'll be accepted and by whom.

If we were to suggest that professionals, particularly teachers and childcare staff, would be willing to condemn a family to hostility, gossip, unkindness, discrimination and isolation, the professionals would be horrified. But they do it. That is what happens today whenever an HIV-positive child (or adult) is denied the right to medical confidentiality.

As a family we are lucky. We have wonderful support from our extended family, our friends, our neighbours, our church and the medical and nursing staff both locally and at the hospital. The exceptions are painful, but fortunately they are few. We are very lucky!

The following contribution is from Susie's brother James.

I was 10 years old when we adopted Susie and until then I had been an only child. I had wanted a brother or sister for sometime but I was quite surprised when my parents asked me how I felt about the idea of adoption. I had understood for some time that my Mum couldn't have another child but adoption never really crossed my mind. Before Susie came to us I was told that she carried the Hepatitis B virus and we all had to have a series of injections to protect us. I was also told that if she fell and bled I wasn't to touch her but to fetch an adult.

When she eventually came to live with us I still couldn't grasp the fact that she was going to be my sister.

About 18 months later I was told that Susie had the HIV virus. I didn't know much about HIV apart from its connection with AIDS but that's about all I knew.

Not long after, Susie had to be enrolled at the local playgroup. It all went smoothly until they told us that we had to tell all the children's parents. Then my Mum and Dad decided not to send me to the local secondary school because it was obvious that the whole village would soon know about Susie and they didn't want me to have trouble at school. Two years have passed since then and almost everyone in my class at school knows about Susie but nobody has really said anything bad to me.

I think my parents told me about Susie in the right way because it would of been terrible for me if someone had walked up to me in the street and asked me something about Susie because I wouldn't have known what they were talking about. I don't really think I needed to know about Susie before I was told. I have learned to adjust to living with Susie and all the safety precautions are just a way of life to me and the rest of the family.

I think that people should understand by now that there is no risk to other children as long as the school's First Aid is of a good standard. I don't think that I should need to know if someone with AIDS was in my class at school so why should anyone else need to know?

The following contribution was written by a young man who learnt of his HIV infection eight months previously.

How I feel

I am the younger of two brothers. My mother and father are divorced and both are in the process of re-marriage. My elder brother is at university. I have an unofficially adopted sister who, together with my elder brother, I can share almost all of my personal problems.

I am the only member of my family who is HIV positive, due to an infected Factor VIII transfusion in 1984. Like all haemophiliacs I was tested for HIV infection every six months and was found to be HIV positive about three months after the injection.

At the time I was not told that I was HIV positive because not only was I very young but the future looked gloomy. I was eventually told at the age of sixteen, when I had been made aware of the essential difference between HIV and AIDS, and the consequences of AIDS. I felt my future looked far brighter after realising I had not got AIDS.

When I was told, I was provided with plenty of up-to-date information from both my father and the hospital, which enabled me to learn more of the way other people had coped with being HIV positive and also allowed me to learn more about the HIV virus and its biological implications.

When I found out I was infected I only told a couple of my very close friends and all my family, although I wanted to tell everyone. However, I now realise that this would have been disastrous. Very few people understand AIDS, other than it is in some ways infectious, and this leads to discrimination.

My family, friends, and a few nurses at the hospital provided plenty of friendly support. My brother, however, gave me the best advice, telling me to write everything down, teaching me meditation and showing me how to avoid being over emotional, by accepting what happens and being realistic about my situation.

I have now known of my HIV infection for eight months. At the time there was no sign of the HIV virus still being present. However, recently my immune system has begun to deteriorate, and I am now on several drugs to help increase my resistance to various diseases.

I now have a far more positive outlook on life than I have ever had before. This is probably due to the realisation that there may be a limitation on how much longer I have to live, and I value my life and everything in it far more. It has also made me stronger willed and more determined in everything I do.

The following contribution was made by Jonathan's mother.
We learnt our only child Jonathan was HIV positive six years ago when he was seven years old. First feelings were of shock, followed by anger that it should have been allowed to happen. We experienced a real fear caused by the uncertainty of the future. Every day on waking it seemed as if there was a black cloud hanging over us. At the beginning Jonathan's HIV status was constantly in our minds and even now is not far beneath the surface. Every time our son had a normal minor illness we wondered if it was the start of AIDS.

We soon desperately wanted to know more about HIV and AIDS. Information from the hospital was sparse, if well intentioned. Even now if we want to know about Jonathan's condition we feel we have to ask, although we have recently been assured that we will be told if anything is amiss. This could be a case of what you don't know you don't worry about – which in our case might be judged a good policy. However, this may not be true for all parents. We have always found information from the Haemophilia Society to be factual, helpful and trustworthy.

Initially, the media response to any news about HIV and AIDS was exaggerated and unhelpful. We found ourselves unable to watch or read about HIV because it seemed so depressing.

The strain of being unable to speak freely about HIV is immense. We had problems and difficulties with Jonathan's school, particularly early on, and because those at school and scouts, etc. remain unaware of Jonathan's HIV status we have worries about the safe treatment of any blood spillages.

As a couple, we have found it difficult to discuss this matter because neither of us wishes to upset the other. Soon after learning of Jonathan's status, when the situation was most difficult, it had an effect on normal communication and consequently was a strain on our relationship. After six years, it can still be difficult to talk to each other about HIV. We feel it would have been very helpful all the way through to have a third party to talk to, either separately or together, preferably detached from the hospital.

The future holds its own dilemma. Like any family, we plan how we would like things to happen in years to come, but you find yourself suddenly thinking if these events will include our son. Irrational, but that's how it is.

As time passes and Jonathan remains well we build up hope and the problems and the worries seem less. We have different views on how things will pan out. It seemed inevitable that our son would eventually get AIDS, but now I refuse to believe this and I feel much more positive and encouraged about the future. I try to live one day at a time and to get my priorities right and to appreciate all the goods things in life. My husband finds this more difficult to accept and sees future hopes fragile and too easily dashed.

The feelings and thoughts of a foster mother.
I am a lone parent in my thirties with a 10-year-old daughter, and I am a foster mother. I am interested in the implications of HIV and AIDS for children in care and their carers.

When I decided to write this piece I thought I knew exactly what I would say – but how wrong I was! I have been caring for an eighteen-month-old boy since his birth, and hopefully adoptive parents will be found soon. He was born to a mother who is HIV positive and whilst he has antibodies, he is a beautiful and healthy baby. I am one of very few people aware of his HIV status and, because he is in care the social workers involved and his specialist doctor also know that he may grow up with HIV. There is a strong bond between the child and myself, and it is hard to believe that he may not grow into a strong and active little boy. I feel very sad at times, realising that not only will he have to endure medical checks, but that one day he may die. In the meantime I realise that it is a great privilege to care for him.

In our family we also have other foster children, none of whom know of the baby's HIV status. We talk freely about AIDS and HIV, together with the subjects of safer-sex and condoms, especially with the older foster children. I know that if they knew of the baby's HIV status they would be disbelieving and then devastated.

I feel as if I have been torn in two by the advice given to me by the social workers, who feel that the information about his HIV status should be kept totally confidential, and the doctor, who feels that all those who are involved in the care (medical and otherwise) should be informed that he carries HIV antibodies. We go to the hospital regularly for check-ups and, although he still carries the antibodies, the results show now that they are less and we hope that one day he will be free of the virus, although we don't known when that will be.

During the past year I have had other foster children who have stayed with us for varying periods of time. Recently I was asked by another local authority to take three children from another family. The alternative was for the children to be separated. They had already been taken into a children's home for their protection and in their best interest. The children are of mixed race, and a suitable home was being sought for them. After some thought I agreed to take the children, aged two, three and five years. Two of the children are HIV positive and one is symptomatic.

The day they arrived was not an easy one for various reasons. The eldest, cautious at first, was soon reassured, especially on finding the toys and his bed. The youngest child was recovering from a head injury, called every one 'Mummy' and cried a lot – he was very withdrawn and looked pale and tired. The three-year-old child gave me great cause for concern. He arrived with a discharging ear which was very smelly, his glands were poking out from his neck like marbles, his abdomen was hard and swollen and his bowels did not open for four days. He was wearing nappies and had bad eczema covering his whole body which was sore and bleeding. He didn't speak, just grunted, and his teeth were rotten. All the children had rotten teeth and their gums were sore.

I had great support from the hospital, and with other help at home – there were seven children in all – we spent the next month growing together in a happy family unit.

The eldest became more cheerful and open – less of a Dad to the others, and more brotherly. The little one became very attached to me – we went for regular visits to the doctor concerning his head injury. He was happy but still confused. The middle child had come a long way. His skin has cleared, he is now potty trained, and talking – does he talk! There is no stopping him. The day he had a haircut he smiled at me and said, 'Mum, don't I look great.'

Soon after the first month I had a call from the social workers who, for various reasons to do with policy, told me these three little boys could not stay. There were problems because they were of mixed race, and I was caring for more children than I had originally agreed to. The boys returned to their own local authority's residential care unit and are now awaiting placements, with the possibility of being separated.

My feelings are of sadness and anger. I was prepared to go to great lengths to help, yet because the policies and guidelines of local authorities are different, we were not able to continue the challenge and enjoyment we had hoped to achieve as a family.

However, I am still caring for the first foster child mentioned above – he is growing well and showing no signs of any illness. I realise it may be difficult to find a long-term home for him and we live with the knowledge that we may care for him indefinitely. There is a great deal of doubt and fear surrounding HIV and AIDS. Foster parents and children alike will benefit greatly from as much support and encouragement as possible.

Appendix

Resource list of organisations and groups

Helplines

BHAN (Black HIV-AIDS Network)
Information, counselling, training and support. A
voluntary group of Asian, African and Afro-Caribbean
men and women.

Tel: 071 485 6756

Black Lesbian and Gay Centre Project

Tel: 081 885 3543
Thursday evening
6pm–9pm.

Body Positive

Tel: 071 373 9124 (helpline)
7pm–10pm daily.

Childline
Support, advice and counselling for children and young
people in trouble or danger.

Tel: 0800 1111 (freephone)

Deaf and Hard of Hearing (VISTEL)

Tel: 071 405 2463
7pm–10pm daily.

Friend
Advice helpline for lesbians and gay men.

Tel: 071 837 3357
7.30pm–10.30pm daily.
Tel: 071 837 2782
Womens line
Thursday evenings.

Jewish Lesbian and Gay Helpline

Tel: 071 706 3123
7pm–10pm Monday and
Thursday.

Legal Line
Advice on legal issues affecting people with HIV, ARC
and AIDS.

Tel: 071 405 2381
7pm–10pm Wednesday
only.

Mainliners
Support and advice for drug users and ex-users.

Tel: 071 274 4000 extn. 354
or 071 738 7333
4pm–9pm daily.

**National AIDS helplines – free and confidential
phonelines**

Tel: 0800 567 123
24 hours

Cantonese and Mandarin AIDS helpline.

Tel: 0800 282 446
Tuesday evenings
6pm–10pm.

Asian AIDS helpline. Advice given in Urdu, Hindi,
Punjabi, Gujerati and Bengali.

Tel: 0800 282 445
Wednesday evenings
6pm–10pm.

Advice given in Arabic.

Tel: 0800 282 4476
6pm–10pm Wednesday
only.

People with hearing disabilities (Minicom)

Tel: 0800 521 361
10am–10pm.

Nurses Support Group
Helpline for healthcare workers who need advice and
help on HIV problems.

Tel: 071 708 5605
7pm–10pm Monday and
Wednesday.

Samaritans
Listed under Samaritans in local telephone directory.

24 hours a day.

**SPOD (Sexual and Personal Relationships of People
with a Disability)**
Counselling for sexual difficulties relating to disability,
including people affected by HIV/AIDS.

Tel: 071 607 8851/2

Survivors
Advice, support and counselling for men who have
been sexually assaulted.

Tel: 071 833 3737

Terrence Higgins Trust
Helpline, information and counselling.

Tel: 071 242 1010 (helpline)
3pm–10pm daily.

Westminster Drugs Project

Tel: 071 286 3339

Grant giving groups

ACET (AIDS Care Education and Training)
National charity, offering home support as well as
financial grants.

PO Box 1323
London W5 5TF
Tel: 081 840 7879

Body Positive
A self help group for people with HIV, ARC and AIDS
who can provide small grants to people with HIV.
Applications should be made in writing.

PO Box 493
London W14 0TF
Tel: 071 835 1045

CHART (Customers Helping AIDS Relief Trust)
Fundraising group which can help people with small
grants.

PO Box 2236
London W14 9EW
Tel: 071 381 1731
Contact: Gerard Bowey

CRUSAID
Fundraising organisation which can help people with
AIDS in need of financial assistance.

21a Upper Tachbrook
Street
London SW1 1SN
Tel: 071 834 7566

LEAN
Small one-off grants available to people in East
London.

PO Box 243
London E6 3H
Tel: 071 473 1534

Mainliners
Gives grants to drug users and ex-users who have
financial problems. Applications must be in writing
with a letter of referral.

PO Box 125
London SW9 8EF
Tel: 071 274 4000 extn. 354

Terrence Higgins Trust
The trust has a hardship fund for people with AIDS.

52–54 Grays Inn Road
London WC1X 8JU
Tel: 071 831 0330

Robert Grace Trust
Small grants available.

Referrals through
Middlesex Hospital

The MacFarlane Trust
For families affected by haemophilia and HIV/AIDS.

PO Box 627
London SW1 0QP
Tel: 071 233 0342
2pm–5pm daily.

Children's organisations

Aberlour Trust
Support group and creche for women and their
children. Advice and residential accommodation.

36 Park Terrace
Stirling FK8 2JR
Tel: 0786 50335
Contact: Joy Roulston

Barnardo's – Positive Options
Information and support for parents with HIV who
need help in planning the future for their children.

354 Goswell Road
London EC1
Tel: 071 278 5039
Contact: Carol Lindsay
Smith

British Youth Council
A national forum for young people in Britain. Produces
excellent resources for training in anti-sexist, anti-racist
work, etc.

57 Charlotte Street
London NW1 1HU
Tel: 071 387 7559

The Children's Legal Centre
Advice service 2pm–5pm weekdays. An advocate for
the rights of children and young people.

20 Compton Terrace
London N1 2UN
Tel: 071 359 6251

Contact-a-Family
An umbrella organisation for numerous parent's
groups.

16 Strutton Ground
London SW1
Tel: 071 222 2695

Department of Education and Science
Produces two leaflets: *Children at School and Problems
Related to AIDS* (no longer published but schools
should have copies); and *AIDS – Some Questions and
Answers – Facts for Teachers, Lecturers and Youth
Workers*.

Publications Despatch
 Centre
Canons Park
London HA7 1AZ

**National Association for the Welfare of Children in
Hospital (NAWCH)**

Argyle House
29–31 Euston Road
London NW1 2SD
Tel: 071 833 2041

**National Association of Young People's Counselling and
Advisory Services (NAYPCAS)**
Offers information and access (by post only) to a
network of youth counselling agencies and annual
training workshops.

17–23 Albion Street
Leicester LE1 6GD

National Childminding Association
Publishes a leaflet 'Who minds about AIDS?' which has
useful information for parents, babysitters and
childminders.

8 Masons Hill
Bromley BR2 9EY
Tel: 081 464 6164

National Children's Bureau

8 Wakely Street
London EC1 7QG
Tel: 071 278 9441

National Foster Care Association
Produces a booklet for carers 'AIDS and HIV –
Information for Foster Parents', which covers most
things which need to be considered when caring for
other people's children.

Francis House
Francis Street
London SW1P 1DE
Tel: 071 828 6266

New Grapevine
Advice and information for young people

416 St John Street
London EC1V 4NJ
Tel: 071 278 9147
(2.30pm–6.30pm)

Parent's Lifeline
Support for parents of critically ill children in hospital.

Tel: 071 263 2265
(24 hour crisis line)

Save The Children Fund

Mary Datchelor House
17 Grove Lane
Camberwell
London SE5 8RD
Tel: 071 703 5400

SOLAS (HIV/AIDS Resource Centre)
Drop-in centre. Support and information for mothers
and children.

2–4 Abbeymount
Edinburgh EH8 8EJ
Tel: 031 661 0982

UNICEF

55 Lincolns Inn Fields
London WC2A 3NB
Tel: 071 405 5592

Voluntary Council for Handicapped Children
A consortium of voluntary and professional
organisations with a broad interest in children with
disability, illness and special needs. It has an extensive
information service.

8 Wakely Street
London EC1V 7QG
Tel: 071 278 9441

An A–Z guide to advice, support and information

ACET (AIDS Care Education and Training)
National charity, offering home support, e.g. home
helps, babysitting, equipment.

PO Box 1323
London W5 5TF
Tel: 081 840 7879

AIDS Ahead
A consortium of organisations for deaf people
supported by the Terrence Higgins Trust, to combat
AIDS. Services include information, counselling and
interpreters.

c/o Cheshire Society for the
Deaf
144 London Road
Northwich
Cheshire CW9 5HH
Tel: 0606 47047

AIDS and Housing Project
Aims to help housing organisations provide good
quality accommodation for people with AIDS, ARC,
HIV.

16–18 Strutton Ground
London SW1P 2HP
Tel: 071 222 6932
Mon–Fri 10am–6pm.

AIDS Support Group
Meetings every other Wednesday at James Pringle
House, London W1. For people with AIDS and their
partners.

Tel: 071 831 0330
Contact: Nick Partridge

AVERT (AIDS Virus Education, Research and Training
An organisation aiming to prevent the spread of AIDS
via education and booklets, etc.

PO Box 91
Horsham
West Sussex RH13 7YR
Tel: 0403 864010

BHAN (Black HIV/AIDS Network)
Black is understood in the widest sense, i.e. people
from non-white backgrounds. Information, counselling
and support.

Tel: 081 741 9565
Mon–Fri 9am–5pm
Contact: Hong Tan

Body Positive
A self help group for anyone who has HIV, ARC or
AIDS. They run a range of groups and courses and a
telephone counselling line which is staffed by people
who have had a positive test or who have AIDS or
ARC. Body Positive can also provide financial help.
Drop-in Centre. Including young people positive group
– 18 to 23 and a womens core group.

51b Philbeach Gardens
Earls Court
London SW5 9EB
Tel: 071 835 1045

Also at
Birmingham
Tel: 021 666 6496

Body Positive Women's Core Group
Support for women affected by HIV.

Shoreditch House
239 Old Street
London EC1
Tel: 071 490 1225
(answerphone)

Brook Advisory Centres (National)
The birth control advice and supplies to young people,
counselling and pregnancy testing.

Central Offices and
enquiries
153a East Street
London SE17 2SD
Tel: 071 708 1234

Buddy Service
Buddies are trained volunteers available to help people
with ARC or AIDS. The service covers house work,
shopping, hospital visiting, advice, information and a
listening ear. Buddies are carefully trained and their
work is intended to complement statutory services, not
substitute them.

c/o Terrence Higgins Trust
52–54 Grays Inn Road
London WC1X 8JU
Tel: 071 831 0330

Citizens Advice Bureaux
National Association of – Help, advice and
information. Look in local telephone directories.

Middleton House
115–123 Pentonville Road
London N1 9LZ
Tel: 081 833 2181 extn. 252/
253

CARA
Care and resources for people affected by AIDS/HIV.
Christian group offering support to Christians or non-
Christians affected by AIDS/HIV.

178 Lancaster Road
London W11 2UU
Tel: 071 792 8299

Catholic AIDS Link
Offer non-judgemental spiritual, emotional and
practical support.

Tel: 081 986 0807
evenings

Childline (see under helplines)

Christian Action on AIDS
A pressure group with representation from all Christian
denominations which encourages churches to adopt
non-judgemental attitudes to people with HIV. Can
give information about churches sympathetic to people
with HIV.

PO Box 74
Hereford HR1 1JX
Tel: 0432 268167
London Tel: 071 476 1505

Cruse Bereavement Care
National organisation with counselling and practical
support for those who have been bereaved.

126 Sheen Road
Richmond
Surrey TW9 1UR
Tel: 081 940 4818

**Foundation for AIDS Counselling, Treatment and
Support (FACTS)**
A medical charity which provides counselling, support
and medical treatment for people with HIV. Their aim
is to enable people to stay at home and be cared for in
the community. FACTS also provide advice for health
professionals such as GPs.

Between 23–25 Weston
Park
Crouch End
London N8 9SY
Tel: 081 348 9195

Families Anonymous
Self-help groups for families affected by drug abuse.

Tel: 071 431 3537

Family Planning Clinics
Local clinics providing information, advice, counselling
and supplies. See local telephone directory.

Family Support Network
This network is for the relatives of people with HIV/
AIDS and of people who have died of ARC or AIDS.
The network offers a monthly support group, home
visits and telephone contact with other members.

c/o Terrence Higgins Trust
Tel: 071 831 0330

The Food Chain
Provides Sunday lunch for people with HIV/AIDS.

Tel: 081 801 4286

Haemophilia Society
The society can supply help and advice for
haemophiliacs, their partners, families and friends.

123 Westminster Bridge
Road
London SE1 7HR
Tel: 071 928 2020
9am–5pm Monday to
Friday.

Haemophilia Support Group
See London Lighthouse and local Haemophilia
Centres.

Health Education Authority

Hamilton House
Mabledon Place
London WC1H 9TX
Tel: 071 383 3833

Immunity
Provides full legal service for people with HIV,
including representation in court. Also produces
publications on legal, medical and civil rights issues.

260 Kilburn Lane
London W10 4BE
Tel: 081 968 8909
10am–5pm Monday to
Friday.

Jewish AIDS Trust
Support, counselling and practical help to people
affected by HIV in the Jewish community.

PO Box 799
London N3 3PN
Tel: 081 455 6449

Kobler Centre
A purpose built out-patient and day-care facility run by
Riverside Health Authority for people with HIV.

St Stephen's Clinic
369 Fulham Road
London SW10 9HT
Tel: 081 846 6161/2
Monday to Friday
9am–5pm

Landmark
A walk-in centre for Lambeth and South London.
Social centre and resource for people with AIDS/HIV
carers, community workers and anyone concerned
about HIV. Advice, transport service, support groups
for men and women.

47a Tulse Hill
London SW2 2TN
Tel: 081 678 6687

LEAN (London East AIDS Network)
A voluntary group for East London. Befriending
service, advice, information and counselling.

PO Box 243
London E6 3HL
Tel: 071 473 1534
(answerphone)

Legal Line
For people with HIV who have legal problems, run by
the Terrence Higgins Trust.

Tel: 071 405 2381
7pm–10pm Wednesday
evenings.

London Lighthouse
Residential and support centre for people with HIV, ARC and AIDS. It aims to offer a range of services to people affected by AIDS including day care counselling, health programmes, training, domiciliary support, respite and terminal care. Support is also provided to partners, friends and families of people with HIV, ARC or AIDS and to those working in the statutory and voluntary services. Drop-in centre and café.

111/117 Lancaster Road
London W11 1QT
Tel: 071 792 1200
Monday to Friday
8.30am–7pm
Saturday and Sunday
12.30pm–4pm

Lovers Support Group
A weekly support group for partners of people who have HIV or AIDS.

c/o Terrence Higgins Trust
Tel: 071 831 0330

Mainliners
Support and advice for people with HIV or AIDS who are drug users, ex-users or maintained users. They offer practical advice on daily living and one to one counselling.

PO Box 125
London SW9 8EF
Tel: 071 274 4000 extn. 354

Manchester AIDS Line
Provides practical and supportive help and has a hardship fund.

Tel: 061 839 2442

Mansfield Settlement
The Mansfield Settlement offers evening meals on Wednesdays for anyone affected by HIV, ARC or AIDS, including carers. Come and enjoy good food and good company. Please ring at least 24 hours in advance. Mainly for people in East London.

Tel: 071 476 1505

Mildmay Mission Hospital
Independent Christian charity providing residential and day care for people with AIDS and for young disabled people. The accent of the unit is on living and enhancing the quality of life.

Hackney Road
London E2 7NA
Tel: 071 739 2331
Homecare team
Tel: 071 729 3616

National Council for One Parent Families
Free advice on law, housing, support services, etc.

255 Kentish Town Road
London NW5 2LX
Tel: 071 261 1361

Needle Exchange
Informal walk-in service from Monday to Friday noon–5.30pm. Offers free needles, condoms, information and counselling.

16A Cleveland Street
London W1 5FD
Tel: 071 631 1750

New Grapevine
Advice and information for young people. Helpline on Tuesdays 10am–2pm and Wednesdays 2pm–6pm. Drop-in on Tuesdays and Wednesdays 2.30pm–6.30pm.

416 St John Street
London EC1V 4NJ
Tel: 071 278 9147

NOVOAH
For information on all voluntary agencies working with AIDS/HIV in the UK.

PO Box 5000
Glasgow G12 9BC
Tel: 041 357 3789
(answerphone)

PACE (Project for Advice Counselling and Education)
Runs training courses and provides one to one
counselling for people with HIV.

London Lesbian and Gay
Centre
67–69 Cowcross Street
London EC1M 6BP
Tel: 071 251 2689
Monday to Friday
9am–5pm

Positively Women
For all women who have HIV, ARC or AIDS. Provides
support counselling and advice for women in and out of
London. Has a fund for HIV-positive women with
children.

c/o Terrence Higgins Trust
Tel: 071 831 0330

Positive Young Gay Group
A support and social group for young (under 25) gay
men who are HIV positive in North London.

Tel: 071 359 2884
Tuesday 6pm–8pm and
answerphone.

Rape Crisis Centre
London contact for a national network of helplines and
support groups for girls and women who have been
raped or sexually assaulted.

Tel: 071 837 1600
24 hour service

Relate (Marriage Guidance Council)
Counselling to *anyone* experiencing problems in a
relationship. Look in local phone books under *Relate*.

National Office
Tel: 0788 73241
Monday to Friday 9am–
5pm

SAM (Scottish AIDS Monitor)
Comprehensive practical help and support. Also has an
office in Glasgow.

64 Broughton Street
Edinburgh EH1 3SA
Tel: 031 557 3885

Samaritans
Organisation to befriend the despairing and suicidal.

National Office
Tel: 0753 32713

SCODA (Standing Conference on Drug Abuse)
Contact the HIV information officer for details of
services and up to date list of needle exchange schemes.

1–4 Hatton Place
London EC1N 8ND
Tel: 071 430 2341

Streetwise
Day centre for people involved in prostitution,
primarily for boys and men up to the age of 21. The aim
is to assist people in their options in or out of
prostitution. Provides support, advice, counselling and
practical help such as baths, washing machine and hot
meals.

Tel: 071 272 8860

Survivors
Gives support and advice on male rape and sexual
assault to victims, their family and friends. Face to face
and telephone advice.

Tel: 071 833 3737
7pm–10pm
Sunday–Friday

Terrence Higgins Trust
Largest HIV charity set up to inform, advise and help
people with HIV and related conditions. Services
include telephone and face to face counselling, welfare
advice, library and information service, health
education and support groups.

52–54 Grays Inn Road
London WC1X 8JU
Tel: 071 831 0330

Turning Point
National network of support centres for drug users,
their relatives and friends.

9–12 Long Lane
London EC1A 9HA
Tel: 071 606 3947

WHRRIC (Womens Health and Reproductive Rights Information Centre)
An information and resource centre on women's health issues. WHRRIC produces information sheets on topics such as 'Women and AIDS' and 'Women and Donor Insemination'.

52–54 Feastherstone Street
London EC1Y 8RT
Tel: 071 251 6332
Mon to Fri 10am–6pm

Women's Support Group
This is a friendly, informal group for women who have had a positive result or who have AIDS. It meets weekly in Central London.

c/o Terrence Higgins Trust
Tel: 071 831 0330

Young People's Positive Group
Self-help information and support for teenagers and young people.

51B Philbeach Gardens
London SW5 9EB
Tel: 071 835 1045
Contact: Anthony Hewitt

Index